Tinnitus and Sound Sensitivity Casebook

Suzanne H. Kimball, AuD, CCC-A, F-AAA
Associate Professor and Undergraduate Program Coordinator
College of Allied Health
University of Oklahoma Health Sciences Center
Oklahoma City, Oklahoma, USA

Marc Fagelson, PhD, CCC-A, F-AAA
Professor of Audiology
Department of Audiology & Speech Pathology
East Tennessee State University
Johnson City, Tennessee, USA

49 Illustrations

Thieme
New York • Stuttgart • Delhi • Rio de Janeiro

Library of Congress Cataloging-in-Publication Data is available from the publisher.

Important note: Medicine is an ever-changing science undergoing continual development. Research and clinical experience are continually expanding our knowledge, in particular our knowledge of proper treatment and drug therapy. Insofar as this book mentions any dosage or application, readersmay rest assured that the authors, editors, and publishers have made every effort to ensure that such references are in accordance with **the state of knowledge at the time of production of the book.**

Nevertheless, this does not involve, imply, or express any guarantee or responsibility on the part of the publishers in respect to any dosage instructions and forms of applications stated in the book. **Every user is requested to examine carefully** the manufacturers' leaflets accompanying each drug and to check, if necessary in consultation with a physician or specialist, whether the dosage schedules mentioned therein or the contraindications stated by the manufacturers differ from the statements made in the present book. Such examination is particularly important with drugs that are either rarely used or have been newly released on the market. Every dosage schedule or every form of application used is entirely at the user's own risk and responsibility. The authors and publishers request every user to report to the publishers any discrepancies or inaccuracies noticed. If errors in this work are found after publication, errata will be posted at www.thieme.com on the product description page.

Some of the product names, patents, and registered designs referred to in this book are in fact registered trademarks or proprietary names even though specific reference to this fact is not always made in the text. Therefore, the appearance of a name without designation as proprietary is not to be construed as a representation by the publisher that it is in the public domain.

Thieme addresses people of all gender identities equally. We encourage our authors to use gender-neutral or gender-equal expressions wherever the context allows.

Thieme Medical Publishers, Inc.
333 Seventh Avenue, 18th Floor,
New York, NY 10001, USA
www.thieme.com
+1 800 782 3488, customerservice@thieme.com

Cover design: Thieme Publishing Group
Cover image source: piano: © Robert Ruidl/stock.adobe.com
(audiogram: © Thieme)
Typesetting by TNQ Technologies, India

Printed in Germany by Beltz Grafische Betriebe   5 4 3 2 1

ISBN: 978-1-68420-167-9

Also available as an e-book:
eISBN (PDF): 978-1-68420-168-6
eISBN (epub): 978-1-63853-684-0

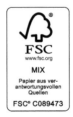

FSC
www.fsc.org
MIX
Papier aus ver-
antwortungsvollen
Quellen
FSC® C089473

Contents

Section A: Medical Cases

I. Tinnitus

Contents

II. Disorders of Sound Tolerance

Foreword

As a health care provider working with patients who present with complaints of tinnitus and/or sound intolerance, you are well aware of the diverse and complex needs of these patients. You are also acutely aware of the lack of resources available to assist us in providing the appropriate clinical services. In the recent years, we have seen an explosion in the literature addressing tinnitus, primarily, and to a lesser extent sound intolerance. Yet, there still is a lack of sufficient evidence-based research to support specific diagnostic assessments and management options related to tinnitus, and even less for sound-intolerance issues.

Perhaps the lack of evidence-based practice and solid research findings on outcomes for managing tinnitus and/or sound intolerance accounts for its lack of inclusion in academic curriculums. Many academic programs cover the topic of tinnitus (and perhaps sound intolerance) in a few lectures, and a few programs have an entire course dedicated to the topic. Henry, Sonstroem, Smith, and Grush (2021) reported that according to their survey of academic programs (32/75 programs participated), all the programs who responded provide training in tinnitus management. Yet, the survey was not an in-depth one so it is not known to what extent each program defined its academic preparation and clinical experience. In addition, it is possible that only programs offering sufficient academic and clinical training in the area of tinnitus responded as the response rate was less than one-half of the programs.

Although we continue to lack in academic preparation and clinical resources, it is improving. In 2017, the Council on Academic Accreditation in Audiology and Speech-Language Pathology (CAA) included tinnitus in their standards for the first time. This should drive increased inclusion of training in this area as academic programs continue to review and update their curricula. In the meantime, practicing clinicians need resources to support their clinical preparation in order to provide best services to their patients/consumers.

This book is an exquisite contribution to expanding the academic and clinical improvements needed in this area. Creating a resource such as this compilation of case studies—illustrating how it is done clinically—is a useful tool for both academic preparation and for the practicing clinician. Each case study demonstrates a unique complexity associated with tinnitus. The inclusion, as opposed to the exclusion, of a related but still independent symptom of sound intolerance further expands the book's usefulness. Many clinicians feel comfortable working with patients with tinnitus. This is especially the case now that so many hearing aid manufacturers offer combination units and their own priority tinnitus management programs. Yet, far fewer feel the same comfort in working with sound-intolerance issues—as the evidence supporting assessment and management is sorely lacking.

The case studies span across both pediatric and adult patients. There are a total of 29 cases included by over 24 authors. These are divided into sections on medical cases, psychological correlates, and legal considerations.

In my review of a number of the case studies, I found each one not only interesting but incredibly educational. Although I have been working with patients with bothersome tinnitus for over 20 years, I found each case offering a pearl that will raise my skill level as a clinician and push me to think outside my clinical box. The design of each case presentation gives the opportunity to solve problem, create your own solution, or provide your expert opinion before launching into a discussion about each one of the questions posed. Each discussion provides the evidence to support the author's opinion and/or actions for additional testing. I especially appreciate the diversity of the cases and the uniqueness of the inclusion of several more challenging cases. In fact, they include cases which could be considered "not successful" or treatment failure as opposed to the typical "textbook" cases.

Overall, I am so very honored to be asked to write this foreword, but more importantly, I am so excited about the publication of this book. It should become a supplementary textbook for every graduate course in the area of tinnitus and sound intolerance, and for those who are already practicing clinicians who provide services to this population of patients, it should become a book that is easily accessible and at your fingertips. I extend my deepest gratitude to Drs. Suzanne H. Kimball and Marc Fagelson for having the idea for this book and seeing it to fruition. The profession of audiology will be elevated because of their efforts as they have provided further evidence of the autonomous but interdisciplinary practice of our profession as we strive to provide the highest level of care to our patients.

Sharon A. Sandridge, PhD
VP
ASHA Audiology Practice;
Section Head
Allied Hearing, Speech and Balance Services
Head and Neck Institute, Cleveland Clinic
Ohio, USA

Preface

Most audiologists would agree that the evaluation and treatment of patients with chronic tinnitus and sound sensitivities can be quite challenging. Clinicians may find that the time needed to adequately and efficiently manage such patients is hard to come by in a busy clinical practice. Others may feel inadequately trained to manage patients who suffer from chronic tinnitus and sound sensitivities as these patients are generally known to be more arduous than a typical patient seen in a hearing clinic. Tinnitus is reported in close to 1 out of every 10 people in the United States alone, and tinnitus-related disabilities are considered some of the most common chronic conditions reported.[1] This prevalence data is similar worldwide. Audiologists may find themselves in a situation where managing these patients is part of their daily clinical routine. It is likely that an equal number of patients with these conditions present to a clinic as those seeking amplification for hearing loss. Patients with tinnitus and sound intolerances often need more help than just hearing aids alone in terms of intervention. Giving support to the field audiologist in the trenches was the impetus for this book.

Dr. Marc Fagelson and I started from the ground up with this collection of tinnitus and sound sensitivity cases several years back. We were solidly into the preproduction of the collection when the CoVID-19 pandemic began. Once the darkest days of the pandemic had passed and we began seeing patients in our clinics again, we quickly came to realize how important such a collection of case studies may be to practicing clinicians, both new and seasoned, as well as to students who may have missed valuable clinical experiences after their clinical placements shut down. In addition, there has been an uptick in patients reporting newly onset and exacerbated preexisting tinnitus post diagnosis of CoVID-19. In other words, the chance that more patients will report to audiology practitioners in the near future is growing even as CoVID-19 vaccinations reach a greater proportion of the population.

The cases herein have been separated into two general categories, namely, tinnitus and sound sensitivities, and are further sorted into medical and psychological segments. Each includes a thorough description of the patient, with most including audiometric test results. Final patient outcomes are provided when available. Readers should note the section titled "Self-Efficacy Considerations" as this section highlights the general takeaway from each case, as well as suggestions to support provision of clinical services. References and Suggested Readings have also been provided. Of special note is that not all cases were written by clinical audiologists; several cases were provided by clinical psychologists. Audiologists should strive to establish professional connections with the mental health specialist community as many patients with chronic tinnitus and sound sensitivities require additional support outside the scope of audiology practice. It behooves an audiologist to establish relationships with local mental health providers, especially if patients with tinnitus and sound sensitivities show significant and life-threatening distress.

I personally established a tinnitus clinic almost a decade ago at the university speech and hearing center where I teach and supervise graduate students. This was done out of a great need which stemmed from lack of resources in our community and across our rural state for patients with tinnitus and sound sensitivities. Patients have literally flocked to our clinic as many patients with these conditions have been ignored or misguided by the medical, audiological, and/or online communities. Many of our patients are desperate, mainly to be "heard" by a practitioner, and to be guided through management with sound science and principles. The goal of this book is to do the same and help guide the practitioners navigate the challenges of tinnitus and sound sensitivity.

Indeed, guiding patients with tinnitus, hyperacusis, or misophonia through the evaluation and treatment process can be difficult. Proper training in tinnitus evaluation and management is essential. Seeing patients with these conditions successfully manage their symptoms has been one of the greatest accomplishments of my professional career. I hope you enjoy reviewing these cases as much as Dr. Fagelson and I enjoyed editing them.

I cannot end this preface without acknowledging many people. First, I want to thank the many hundreds of tinnitus and sound sensitivity patients I have seen throughout the years; my teaching, research, and clinical pursuits have all been because of wanting the best for each of you. To the many students

I have taught over my decades in the university setting, I hope that I am able to leave a little part of me within each of you, so that my work in the classroom and in the clinic can be carried on for many years to come. My thanks also to my co-editor, Dr. Marc Fagelson, for teaming up with me on this crazy adventure, even in the midst of a pandemic! Thanks to my favorite people in this life, my husband Roger and kids Annette, Jared, and Madeline who are always there to support me with a kind and encouraging word.

My biggest "thank you" goes out to my mom and dad, Rita and Peter, for always believing in me, bragging on my every accomplishment, both big and small, and always calling me their favorite!

I hope you enjoy this collection.

Reference

[1] Bhatt JM, Lin HW, Bhattacharyya N. Prevalence, severity, exposures, and treatment patterns of tinnitus in the United States. JAMA Otolaryngol Head Neck Surg. 2016;142(10): 959–965

Suzanne H. Kimball, AuD, CCC-A, F-AAA

Preface

Patients experiencing bothersome tinnitus and problems related to sound intolerance remain an underserved population, often in need of substantial help from audiologists, psychologists, and physicians. Many academic programs in audiology struggle to provide classroom and clinical opportunities for students to gain experience and confidence working with patients whose conditions may not respond favorably when compared to the more routine interventions practiced in audiology clinics, or covered in audiology classes. This book of cases will not solve the problem. However, it presents reports from clinicians whose experiences provide both enlightening and cautionary tales intended to support patient care, clinicians' self-efficacy, and student learning.

Patients whose cases appear in the text represent some of the more challenging clinical encounters facing hearing health care providers. Sound intolerance comes in many forms, and the text offers several examples of clinicians employing innovative interventions that rely on desensitization and other forms of exposure therapies intended to reduce the patients' powerful aversions to specific sounds and situations. Similarly, the text provides examples of clinical interventions that may be adapted in order to address, in a reasonable manner, patients' reported problems. Several of the chapters contain specific tips for clinicians to consider; these suggestions should support clinicians' certainty, or self-efficacy, regarding their ability to provide for patients. As with any aspect of practice, the onus is on the provider to earn the patient's trust. But this process likely begins with the providers feeling confident about their grasp of the patient's condition, as well as their familiarity with the strategies available as clinical interventions. This text will support the audiologist who needs to understand and help guide the patients' rehabilitation journey when confronted by tinnitus and sound intolerance.

Does the number of patients requiring services for tinnitus and sound intolerance resemble the number of patients who would benefit from hearing aid use? Clearly, audiologists have expressed their choice; many more practitioners appear more willing and able to fit hearing aids than to take on the challenges associated with tinnitus and sound intolerance. Professionally, this situation represents a failure on many levels, from programmatic instruction to the availability of clinical opportunities. Ironically, many individuals seek careers in audiology with the somewhat vague goal of "helping others." Vague though it may be, the notion of reducing others' suffering, in this area of audiology's scope, requires a provider who is willing to learn novel strategies relevant to underserved and often-desperate patients. We hope that exposure to cases provided by active clinicians willing to take on the challenge will help others accept the feasibility of such a practice.

I am grateful for the collaboration required to produce this text. Dr. Suzanne H. Kimball contacted me a few years ago with support from Thieme Publishers. Dr. Kimball steered us through unprecedented circumstances, maintained focus, recruited authors, and somehow found the time to keep her own program's needs met. I've worked closely with her for more than 2 years, and we've still not met in person. For all I know, each time we have spoken, she was sitting in a canoe in her office! During our discussions, we often came back to a point of emphasis: Patients who suffer the most, in many ways, offer the provider the greatest opportunity to help. We hope this modest text will spark interest in, and care for, patients whose needs often go unmet. Come join us in this endeavor, we need you!

Marc Fagelson, PhD, CCC-A, F-AAA

Contributors

David M. Baguley, PhD
Professor in Hearing Sciences
Mental Health and Clinical Neurosciences,
    School of Medicine, University of Nottingham
Nottingham, UK

Christi Barbee, AuD
Associate Professor
University of Oklahoma Health Sciences Center
Oklahoma City, Oklahoma, USA

Erin Benear, AuD, CCC-A
Clinical Assistant Professor–Clinical Coordinator
Department of Communication
    Sciences and Disorders
University of Oklahoma Health Sciences
    Center, College of Allied Health
Oklahoma City, Oklahoma, USA

Eldre Beukes, PhD
Audiologist and Lecturer
Vision and Hearing Sciences Research Centre,
    School of Psychology and Sport Sciences
Anglia Ruskin University
Cambridge, UK

Jennifer Jo Brout, PsyD
Licensed Professional Counselor
JJB Counseling & Consultation, LLD
International Misophonia Research Network
Bay Pines VA Healthcare System
Bay Pines, Florida, USA

Diana Callesano, AuD, CCC-A/FAAA
Audiologist
Hearing and Tinnitus Center
Woodbury, New York, USA

Trevor Courouleau, AuD, CCC-A
Clinical Associate Professor of Audiology
Department of Communication
    Sciences and Disorders
OSU Speech-Language-Hearing Clinic,
    042 Social Sciences and Humanities
Stillwater, Oklahoma, USA

Aniruddha K. Deshpande, PhD, CCC-A
Associate Professor;
Director
The Hear-Ring Lab, Department of
    Speech-Language-Hearing Sciences
Hofstra University
Hempstead, New York, USA

Catherine M. Edmonds, AuD,
  CCC-A, ABA CH-TM
Audiologist
Bay Pines VA Health System
Bay Pines, Florida, USA

Marc Fagelson, PhD, CCC-A, F-AAA
Professor of Audiology
Department of Audiology & Speech Pathology
East Tennessee State University
Johnson City, Tennessee, USA

Isabella Hillerby, BS
Doctor of Audiology Student
Department of Communication Sciences and
    Disorders
College of Allied Health, University of
    Oklahoma Health Sciences Center
Oklahoma City, Oklahoma, USA

Michael Hoffman, PhD
Nemours Children's Health and Assistant
Professor of Pediatrics
Sidney Kimmel Medical College
Thomas Jefferson University
Philadelphia, USA

Wan Syafira Ishak, B. Audiology (Hons), PhD
Senior Lecturer & Audiologist
Audiology Program, Centre for Healthy Ageing
    and Wellness (H-CARE)
Faculty of Health Sciences, Universiti
    Kebangsaan
Kuala Lumpur, Malaysia

Rebecca Jimenez, AuD
USA

Melissa Karp, AuD
Audiologist
Audiology & Hearing Service of Charlotte
Charlotte, North Carolina, USA

Suzanne H. Kimball, AuD, CCC-A, F-AAA
Associate Professor;
Undergraduate Program Coordinator
College of Allied Health, University of
    Oklahoma Health Sciences Center
Oklahoma City, Oklahoma, USA

Christopher Kuykendall, AuD
Audiologist
Mercy Health Systems
Oklahoma City, Oklahoma, USA

Lauren Mann, AuD, PhD
School of Health Professions
Department of Hearing and Speech
University of Kansas Medical Center
Kansas City, Kansas, USA

Don McFerran, MA, FRCS
Consultant ENT Surgeon
East Suffolk and North Essex
    NHS Foundation Trust
Colchester, UK

Jamie Myers, AuD
USA

Colleen A. O'Brien, AuD, CCC-A, F-AAA
Research Audiologist
NYU Grossman School of Medicine, Manhattan
    VA Medical Center
New York, USA

Jenna M. Pellicori, AuD, CCC-A
Nemours Children's Health and Assistant
Professor of Pediatrics
Sidney Kimmel Medical College
Thomas Jefferson University
Philadelphia, USA

Ann Perreau, PhD
Associate Professor of Communication
    Sciences and Disorders;
Audiology Clinic Coordinator
Augustana College
Rock Island, Illinois, USA

Ana Rabasco, MA
Department of Psychology
Fordham University
New York, USA

Tammy Riegner, AuD, CCC-A
Nemours Children's Health and Assistant
Professor of Pediatrics
Sidney Kimmel Medical College
Thomas Jefferson University
Philadelphia, USA

Myles S. Rizvi, PsyD
Licensed Clinical Psychologist;
Senior Clinician
NW Anxiety Institute, NW Anxiety Pediatrics
Portland, Oregon, USA

LaGuinn P. Sherlock, AuD, CH-TM
US Army Public Health Center
Army Hearing Program
Aberdeen Proving Grounds
Aberdeen, Maryland, USA

Jason H. Thomas, Au.D, CCC-A, F-ADA
Clinical Coordinator of Audiology
Adjunct Professor
St. John's University
Queens, New York, USA

Richard S. Tyler, PhD
Professor of Otolaryngology;
Professor of Communication
    Sciences and Disorders
Roy J. and Lucille A. Carver College of Medicine
Department of Otolaryngology – Head and
    Neck Surgery, University of Iowa
Iowa City, Iowa, USA

Section A: Medical Cases

I: Tinnitus

1 Internet-Based Tinnitus Intervention

Eldre Beukes

1.1 Clinical History/Description

Patient A attended his local tinnitus clinic due to distressing tinnitus. He had a mild hearing loss and was not using hearing aids. An initial tinnitus therapy session provided explanations about tinnitus and sleep hygiene. Practically arranging appointments was difficult as he was employed abroad and was not able to attend his local clinic frequently. The clinic suggested registering for a study looking at the effects of an Internet-based tinnitus intervention as this was prior to teleaudiology being frequently used. The patient registered and completed the screening questionnaire. This indicated that he was aged between 40 and 50 years. He had experienced tinnitus constantly for 2 years in both ears. The tinnitus was described as a complex presentation of ringing, buzzing, low and high pitched sounds, pulsating, clicking, music, voices, and humming. He attributed his tinnitus to long periods of exposure to noise without adequate hearing protection. He described being generally grumpy and irritable as a result of the tinnitus. Specific difficulties included trouble getting to sleep, concentrating, and hearing on his mobile phone and the television. Loud noises were annoying and aggravated the tinnitus. Hyperacusis together with tinnitus resulted in him being unable to do the things he previously enjoyed. Although he was struggling to hear, he did not want hearing aids. He explained that he hated anything in his ears.

Both the Tinnitus Functional Index[1] and the Tinnitus Handicap Inventory[2] were administered and indicated a moderate impact of tinnitus with scores of 44/100 and 48/100, respectively. Mild levels of anxiety and depression were identified (8/21 on the Generalized Anxiety Disorder Questionnaire[3]; 5/28 on the Patient Health Questionnaire[4]). The Insomnia Severity Index[5] showed subthreshold insomnia at 10/28. There was mild hearing concerns (14/40 on the Hearing Handicap Inventory[6]). Strong hyperacusis was present (28/40 on the Hyperacusis Questionnaire[7]).

1.2 Questions for the Reader

1. With this level of tinnitus severity, should an Internet-based intervention be considered?
2. By what means should we be evaluating the presence of comorbid conditions for individuals with tinnitus?
3. Beyond those relating to co-occurring conditions, which outcome domains should we be assessing?
4. Which outcome measures should be used to assess intervention-related changes in tinnitus severity?
5. Which other specific outcome measures should we consider for those with tinnitus?

1.3 Discussion of Questions

1. *With this level of tinnitus severity, should an Internet-based intervention be considered?*
   Internet-based interventions have predefined inclusion and exclusion criteria. Generally, a minimum cut-off score for inclusion ensures that participants have the potential to observe benefit from the study intervention; no maximum cut-off score was specified. Internet intervention studies tend to exclude people who have other serious additional health or mental health problems or those who are undertaking additional interventions. A complex range of factors contribute to a successful outcome; however, the factors may not be clear before commencing the intervention. The patient in this case had difficulty attending his local clinic and although he met all inclusionary criteria, he presented with mild levels of anxiety and depression. Such patients require careful monitoring to ensure their ability to complete the intervention, and to determine whether any additional services are required.
2. *By what means should we be evaluating the presence of comorbid conditions?*
   Good justification is required for each assessment measure administered. In an Internet-based intervention there is a greater possibility of not detecting problems as there is no face-to-face interaction with the patient. Although a thorough investigation of symptoms is required, there is also a fine balance between a thorough case history and overloading the patient. If many assessment measures are required, then their selection should consider the effort and fatigue of the patient completing

the forms. Very high levels of anxiety and depression should be identified and may need attending to before the patient is able to focus on addressing the tinnitus (see ▶ Table 1.2 for examples of intake forms).

3. *Beyond those relating to co-occurring conditions, which outcome domains should we be assessing?* This is an important question. There are many possibilities. Some research has looked at specific outcomes that tinnitus patients find are most relevant to them. A Delphi study indicated domains such as concentration, quality of sleep, sense of control, mood, negative thoughts are important to stakeholders.[8] Ideally, a core set of domains assessed across clinics would be ideal. Further work is required to establish the most appropriate and psychometrically robust measures for a tinnitus population. In view of these limitations, work is currently underway to identify a core set of outcome measures for tinnitus.[9,10]

4. *Which outcome measures should be used to assess intervention-related changes in tinnitus severity?* Both the TFI and THI were used here for comparative purposes. The measures selected should address various factors such as the purpose of testing (diagnostics/responsiveness to treatment). It is also important to consider whether the questionnaire is validated psychometrically for the population being tested. The TFI was specifically designed and validated to assess responsiveness to treatment, where many other tinnitus measures were designed for diagnostic purposes only.

5. *Which other specific outcome measures should we consider for those with tinnitus?* ▶ Table 1.2 lists some suggestions. These are not the only options. The considerations mentioned above apply to selecting other questionnaires as well. These have generally been considered as secondary outcome measures. Thus short outcome measures may be preferred.

1.4 Final Diagnosis and Recommended Treatment

The patient was randomized to receive 8 weeks of Internet-based cognitive behavioral therapy (CBT) principles for tinnitus. This intervention consisted of the following key elements[11,12]:

- The intervention was provided on a purpose-built secure web-based platform. It had the required security features in place for data protection.
- The content was based on CBT principles as these presently have the most robust evidence of effectiveness in minimizing the effects of tinnitus, particularly longer-term.[13] Audiological principles formed from clinical experience and research found to be effective for tinnitus also informed the theoretical base of the intervention.
- The content was divided into different modules. Two to three modules were released on a weekly basis with a core of 16 modules recommended to all participants. An additional five modules were optional and only recommended for specific difficulties related to insomnia, concentration, hyperacusis, and communication problems.
- It was a guided intervention with an audiologist who reviewed participants' work and progress. A secure messaging system enabled communication between the audiologist and patients.
- There were interactive elements, such as videos and worksheets, to encourage engagement in the intervention. These could be completed during or outside intervention-related activities.
- The intervention materials were accessible by ensuring they were not difficult to read and no complex terminology was used.

The first module discussed the requirements for the intervention. These included trying to set aside some time each day to work on the strategies suggested. The patient indicated he would work at it each morning before work, but just after breakfast. The module emphasized the commitment required and setting some goal with some suggestions to select. The patient indicated that he was 100% committed and willing to try new things. The specific goals he set were: (i) learning how to cope with the tinnitus more effectively rather than battle with it; (ii) having a better understanding of tinnitus; (iii) making the tinnitus less annoying and intrusive; (iv) being able to relax more easily; and (v) reduce tension and stress caused by work and tinnitus.

1.5 Progress during and after Undertaking the Intervention

The patient was monitored weekly by means of the THI screening version. Results are shown in ▶ Fig. 1.1. It indicates a gradual decline over time

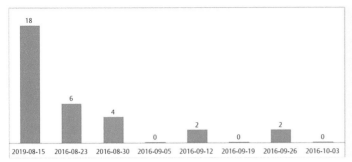

Fig. 1.1 THI-screening scores, measured weekly while doing the intervention. Lower scores indicate less severity.

and that this improvement is maintained. The large initial decline early on between weeks 1 and 2 is substantial and may be related to being on an intervention and knowing he is getting support. It could also be related to the impact of the help from the initial modules.

The modules completed are shown in ▶ Table 1.1. He read all the modules and completed the relevant modules. He was very engaged and regularly logged into the website. ▶ Table 1.2 also provides his usefulness ratings and comments about the modules. Note that the patient found some modules, such as trying to reinterpret his tinnitus, less useful than those covering relaxation.

Following the intervention, the same questionnaires were completed. Improvements were seen on all forms, as shown in ▶ Table 1.2. It is encouraging these improvements were maintained one year later despite no further intervention. The patient found the CBT tools useful as they could be done anywhere. The tools were handy as he spends a lot of time travelling; he reported using many of the strategies during his daily life. For example, when realizing he was getting uptight about something he would remember and employ specific strategies to calm himself down.

As clinical scores do not always relate to patient perceptions, the patient was interviewed about his experiences. He indicated that no further treatment was required. Overall, he found the program very helpful as can be seen from responses in ▶ Table 1.3.

1.6 Questions for the Reader

1. Can treatment be stopped at this point?
2. Why have the scores decreased more at 1-year postintervention?
3. Why have most of the scores decreased, such as hearing disability despite not wearing amplification?

1.7 Discussion of the Questions for the Reader

1. *Can intervention be stopped at this point?*
   Having a set treatment period can be beneficial. The patient knew he was required to commit for 8 weeks and his progress would then be reviewed. Looking at the outcome measure scores alone, the levels indicated are generally below the levels suggesting clinical care is required. It is important also finding out from the patient whether they have achieved their goals and require any further help. He indicated that he had enough strategies to cope and did not require further help.
2. *Why have the scores decreased more at 1-year post-intervention?*
   The intervention period is there to provide the strategies and try them. Following this the patient is likely to continue using the strategies that are most effective. This patient had clearly internalized the strategies and was applying them to different situations in daily life. It is likely that over time they were done without thinking, such as better managing a stressful event which in the past may have triggered his tinnitus to flare-up.
3. *Why have most of the scores decreased, such as hearing disability despite not wearing amplification?*
   The theoretical framework of the intervention is based on CBT. The aim of CBT is to lead to positive behavioral change. If these behavioral changes are made they can have an effect on secondary tinnitus effects, such as the perception that tinnitus impairs hearing. This may not be assessed, as interventions primarily focus on identifying whether tinnitus severity has decreased. It is encouraging to see additional intervention effects.

Table 1.1 Modules undertaken, usefulness score, and comments

Category	Module	Usefulness rating	Patient comments taken from his worksheets
General	Understanding tinnitus	5	I learned the term habituation. It's about getting used to tinnitus. I still focus on it and get stressed over it. New techniques will steer me away from this. I like the example of a new picture on the wall and I can relate to this very well
	Progressive relaxation program (six steps from deep relaxation to rapid relaxation)	5	Good use of positive imagery and a really good session. After tensing muscle groups It feels like I can feel them unwind and I feel much lighter in those areas so hopefully, I have the technique correct
Cognitive behavioral therapy	Reinterpreting tinnitus	2	Can visualize everything well, plant room, closing the door, going up on deck surrounding area, but finding this difficult view as an alternative sound. Will try again for a few days if not then I may have to find a different image
	Positive imagery	5	Snorkeling, able to focus 95%, combined with relaxation, so I dived into the sea first swam around explored a bit, different shoals of fish, the sea bed then did my relaxation exercises and then continued to explore, found a ship wreck a clown fish. This seems to work. It feels like it's working well
	Identifying negative thoughts and cognitive restructuring	4	Don't over think the "what if, why me, If only I had" thoughts anymore It has happened and now we have a method to deal with the tinnitus. The main aim is not to be stressed by tinnitus and to recognize what causes the stress before it happens. Then to relax and everything is easier to accept and deal with. A calm approach helps every time and this can prevent the tinnitus from becoming annoying and its then manageable
	Exposure to tinnitus	4	Reflecting back initially my tinnitus bothered me but toward the end of the session after I had relaxed I sat still for a minute as was unaware of my tinnitus, It felt so good
	Focus	5	Finding it hard to concentrate on only one sound, will keep working at it
Optional modules	Sound enrichment	4	I use different sounds throughout the day when working at my desk. I find one sound it too much
	Sleep guidelines	5	I now get up the same time every day, and go to bed within 1 hour every day, I have reduced caffeinated beverages before bedtime
	Hyperacusis	4	Unload and load the dishwasher alone in the quiet to get used to the noise Low back ground noise when working when alone in the house. This is definitely helping
	Hearing tactics	5	Useful tips to help me hear better. Patisserie-avoid dump waiter area, I usually ask to sit upstairs as downstairs has too many awkward areas, each corner has its problems, 1 toilet area, 2 dumbwaiter area, 3 main door, 4 serving area and people queuing

Note: All the modules were recommended due to his preintervention scores. Usefulness ratings: 1=low; 5=high.

Table 1.2 Postintervention outcomes and 1-y follow-up outcomes

Outcome measures	Abbreviation	Initial score	Postintervention	1-y f/u
Tinnitus Functional Index	TFI[1]	44	9	2
Tinnitus Handicap Inventory	THI[2]	48	18	6
Hearing Handicap Inventory	HHIA[6]	14	6	6
Generalized Anxiety Disorder Questionnaire	GAD-7[3]	8	5	5
Health Questionnaire	PHQ-9[4]	5	1	0
Insomnia Severity	ISI[5]	10	0	0
Satisfaction with Life	SWLS[14]	32	32	33
Hyperacusis	HQ[7]	28	14	11
Cognitive Failures Questionnaire	CFQ[15]	29	21	19

Table 1.3 Comments about the intervention undertaken

Questions asked	Comments
What was the best aspect of your treatment?	Having a structure and positive feedback and advice from the personal messages. It helped me understand and enabled me to adjust and accept the tinnitus and be more relaxed about it
How has it helped?	Thank you for your support throughout, it has helped tremendously and I have such a better understanding, feeling and approach to my tinnitus, these last few weeks it has reduced enormously, with minor flare-ups. I successfully attended to Pantos this year and my tinnitus did not prevent me from having a wonderful time. The stress and relaxing techniques have been wonderful and these will remain part of my daily and weekly routine wherever I may be in the world. The program has helped me relax and reflect differently on tinnitus. I now feel I can cope a lot better with tinnitus
Which modules were the most helpful?	I have found the relaxation technique program very informative and some elements I felt I have really benefited from. Shifting Focus was a hard concept and this I did not get on well with. Whereas positive imagery and the relaxation steps provided me with excellent results. To the extent that I have had a few weeks where my tinnitus has virtually been non-existent. Trying to look at negative thoughts from a different angle has also helped. In general the more relaxed less stressful I am the less my tinnitus flares up
What will you continue using?	I will keep the techniques going as I have seen the benefit of them. I have found over the last month that by trying to keep less stressed has had a huge impact on my tinnitus. I will continue to incorporate all the relaxation techniques, from the deep to the rapid, into my everyday life. By making situations less stressful then it's easier to cope and makes one feel in a better place. Sleep hygiene and routine is a real benefit although extremely difficult when working away, but this is where the rapid techniques help, just before and after a meal. With deeper techniques at bedtimes. I have learned to break my worries down. This makes it much more manageable and achievable, that way I still feel in control and this helps me manage my tinnitus

References

[1] Meikle MB, Henry JA, Griest SE, et al. The tinnitus functional index: development of a new clinical measure for chronic, intrusive tinnitus. Ear Hear. 2012; 33(2):153–176

[2] Newman CW, Jacobson GP, Spitzer JB. Development of the tinnitus handicap inventory. Arch Otolaryngol Head Neck Surg. 1996; 122(2):143–148

[3] Spitzer RL, Kroenke K, Williams JB, Löwe B. A brief measure for assessing generalized anxiety disorder: the GAD-7. Arch Intern Med. 2006; 166(10):1092–1097

[4] Kroenke K, Spitzer RL. The PHQ-9: A new depression diagnostic and severity measure. Psychiatr Ann. 2002; 32(9): 509–515

[5] Bastien CH, Vallières A, Morin CM. Validation of the Insomnia Severity Index as an outcome measure for insomnia research. Sleep Med. 2001; 2(4):297–307

[6] Newman CW, Weinstein BE, Jacobson GP, Hug GA. Test-retest reliability of the hearing handicap inventory for adults. Ear Hear. 1991; 12(5):355–357

[7] Khalfa S, Dubal S, Veuillet E, Perez-Diaz F, Jouvent R, Collet L. Psychometric normalization of a hyperacusis questionnaire. ORL J Otorhinolaryngol Relat Spec. 2002; 64(6):436–442

[8] Hall DA, Smith H, Hibbert A, et al. Core Outcome Measures in Tinnitus (COMiT) initiative. The COMiT'ID study: Developing core outcome domains sets for clinical trials of sound-, psychology-, and pharmacology-based interventions for

chronic subjective tinnitus in adults. Trends in hearing. 2018 Nov;22:2331216518814384

[9] Rademaker MM, Essers BA, Stokroos RJ, Smit AL, Stegeman I. What tinnitus therapy outcome measures are important for patients?–a discrete choice experiment. Frontiers in Neurology. 2021;12

[10] Shabbir M, Akeroyd MA, Hall DA. A comprehensive literature search to identify existing measures assessing "concentration" as a core outcome domain for sound-based interventions for chronic subjective tinnitus in adults. Progress in brain research. 2021 Mar 13;262:209–224

[11] Beukes EW, Vlaescu G, Manchaiah V, et al. Development and technical functionality of an Internet-based intervention for tinnitus in the UK. Internet Interv. 2016; 6:6–15

[12] Beukes EW, Fagelson M, Aronson EP, et al. Readability following cultural and linguistic adaptations of an Internet-based intervention for tinnitus for use in the United States. American Journal of Audiology. 2020 Jun 8;29(2):97–109

[13] Fuller T, Cima R, Langguth B, et al. Cognitive behavioural therapy for tinnitus. Cochrane Database of Systematic Reviews. 2020(1)

[14] Diener E, Emmons RA, Larsen RJ, Griffin S. The satisfaction with life scale. J Pers Assess. 1985; 49(1):71–75

[15] Broadbent DE, Cooper PF, FitzGerald P, Parkes KR. The cognitive failures questionnaire (CFQ) and its correlates. Br J Clin Psychol. 1982; 21(1):1–16

Suggested Readings

Beukes EW, Andersson G, Allen PM, Manchaiah V, Baguley DM. Effectiveness of guided Internet-based cognitive behavioral therapy vs face-to-face clinical care for treatment of tinnitus: a randomized clinical trial. JAMA Otolaryngol Head Neck Surg. 2018; 144(12):1126–1133

Beukes EW, Allen PM, Baguley DM, Manchaiah V, Andersson G. Long-term efficacy of audiologist-guided Internet-based cognitive behavior therapy for tinnitus. Am J Audiol. 2018; 27 3S:431–447

Beukes EW, Manchaiah V, Davies ASA, Allen PM, Baguley DM, Andersson G. Participants' experiences of an Internet-based cognitive behavioural therapy intervention for tinnitus. Int J Audiol. 2018; 57(12):947–954

2 Chiari Malformation with Tinnitus and Hyperacusis

Suzanne H. Kimball

2.1 Clinical History and Description

LO is a 53-year-old female with a history of Chiari malformation treated with decompression surgery in November of 2017. The patient also has a history of head injury, concussion, migraine headaches, motion sickness, and epilepsy. She reported a history of bilateral tinnitus, which was exacerbated during a migraine, as well as hyperacusis, hearing loss, and aural pressure. LO reported that her tinnitus greatly affected her ability to concentrate, sleep, and enjoy quiet recreational activities (all subjectively ranked an 8 out of 10 in severity). During the intake interview, she indicated that her tinnitus was catastrophically affecting her quality of life (ranked a 10/10). In regard to her hyperacusis complaint, she was bothered by loud concerts, movies, restaurants, church services, housekeeping items such as vacuum cleaners, and loud/screaming children. When prompted in the intake interview, LO ranked her tinnitus severity as a 10/10 and her sound intolerance as a 9/10.

LO was originally seen at an otolaryngology practice for an audiological evaluation in April 2018. Results at that time indicated normal hearing sensitivity in the right ear and normal hearing sensitivity through 4000 Hz sloping to a mild hearing loss at 6000 and 8000 Hz in the left ear (see audiogram). She reported prior myringotomy tube placement (for ear pressure) with no perceived benefit. LO was referred to our university speech and hearing clinic due to her bothersome tinnitus, sound sensitivity, and dizziness (▶ Fig. 2.1).

2.2 Audiological Testing

LO experienced several seizures in the days prior to her appointment at our facility. Due to her seizure disorder and the distance from our clinic to her home (roughly 2 h), LO was accompanied by a friend. Because she had completed a hearing evaluation less than 4 months prior to visiting our clinic, a comprehensive audiometric evaluation was not conducted. Tympanometry was performed and indicated bilateral Type A tympanograms, consistent with normal middle ear function for both ears. Pure-tone thresholds were screened to ensure that

no changes in hearing sensitivity had occurred since the time of her prior testing.

2.3 Tinnitus Evaluation

LO completed our clinic tinnitus case history intake form, the Tinnitus Handicap Inventory[1] (THI) and the Tinnitus Functional Index[2] (TFI). She scored an 80 on the THI and an 82% on the TFI. These results suggested that her ability to carry out routine activities and her quality of life were substantially reduced by her tinnitus symptoms.

High-frequency audiometry and uncomfortable loudness testing were conducted (see audiogram). Uncomfortable loudness testing identified slightly reduced loudness tolerance (80–95 dB HL uncomfortable loudness levels [UCLs] from 500 to 4,000 Hz) bilaterally for both speech and pure-tone conditions (▶ Fig. 2.2). A tinnitus evaluation including pitch match, loudness match, minimal masking for wideband noise, and residual inhibition was completed.

During residual inhibition testing, LO experienced a partial seizure (although she did not appear to have full convulsions, she indicated to us that she was having a seizure), during which she lost a few seconds of memory, and experienced increased heart rate, audible heart beats, and "electricity shooting through her veins." We asked LO's friend to join us in the testing suite as she had more experience with LO's seizure episodes and could direct us in how to best assist her. After LO recuperated from the seizure (with a 10–15 min rest period), testing was ended and counseling regarding results and recommendations commenced.

2.4 Questions for the Reader

1. What additional case history information might be pertinent to this case?
2. What is Chiari malformation?
3. How is Chiari malformation treated?
4. What other case history information is significant?
5. What management options specific to Chiari could support tinnitus relief?
6. What other medical professionals should be involved in the management of her tinnitus and sound sensitivity?

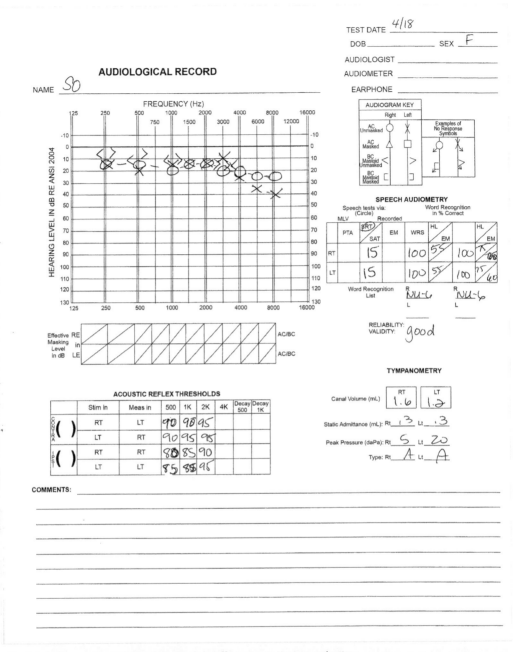

Fig. 2.1 Audiogram generated at otolaryngology office prior to tinnitus evaluation.

2.5 Discussion of Questions for the Reader

1. *What additional case history information might be pertinent to this case?*
   It would be beneficial to determine the nature of LO's seizure disorder and the triggers that

appear to exacerbate it (like the sounds used in the tinnitus evaluation). Perhaps asking the patient whether sounds trigger any form of seizure activity would have been helpful. Audiogenic seizures are convulsions brought on by prolonged exposure to high-frequency sound, but have been researched mostly in

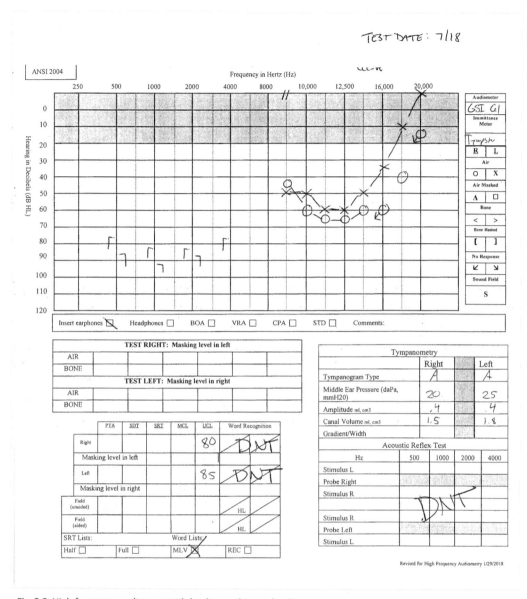

Fig. 2.2 High-frequency audiogram with loudness tolerance levels.

rodents and rabbits. Some evidence suggests that audiogenic seizures in humans are possible, but have not been studied extensively.[3]

2. *What is Chiari malformation?*
   According to the Mayo Clinic, Chiari malformation is a condition in which brain tissue extends into the spinal canal. It occurs when part of the skull is abnormally small or misshapen, pressing on the brain and forcing it downward. There are three categories of Chiari,

which are each classified by the presence and severity of symptoms. Symptoms can range from none to severe but can include tinnitus, hyperacusis, dizziness, weakness, numbness, and more.

3. *How is Chiari malformation treated?*
   Treatment varies depending on the severity but can include surgery. In the most common surgery for Chiari malformation, called posterior fossa decompression, a surgeon removes a small section of bone in the back of the skull, relieving

pressure on the brain and providing the tissue room to expand without constriction.

4. *What other case history information is significant?*

Clearly this patient had a complicated medical history. Her seizures, unsteadiness, and migraines all must be considered in her management. Paulin et al[4] showed that migraine is a risk factor for hyperacusis. In addition, tinnitus and hyperacusis have been reported in a variety of musculoskeletal and neurological illnesses, which may have relevance to this particular patient.[5]

5. *What management options might be considered for tinnitus relief?*

Based on the Jastreboff protocol for Tinnitus Retraining Therapy[6] (TRT), which we utilize at our clinic, tinnitus and hyperacusis can be managed with a systematic program of sound therapy and counseling. The patient is instructed to use sound therapy at a comfortable level, at first to foster desensitization, and then to partially mask but not completely cover the tinnitus. Sound therapy can be introduced through a variety of methods including hearing aids, tinnitus maskers, standalone devices, or smartphone apps. Hyperacusis can be managed with desensitization exercises and sound therapy. In addition, this patient could also benefit from strategies such as relaxation and controlled breathing.

6. *What other medical professionals should be involved in the management of her tinnitus and sound sensitivity?*

Much of this patient's medical issues go far beyond the scope of practice for an audiologist. Her neurologist and pain management doctors were clearly needed as part of her comprehensive management team. In addition, as LO reported a poor quality of life, a referral to a mental health professional would be appropriate.

2.6 Final Diagnosis and Recommended Treatment

In addition to her significant medical history, LO offered another complicating factor. She reported an intolerance to the sensation of "anything in her ears." This aversion limited management options from the standpoint of tinnitus maskers, amplification devices, or standalone sound therapy devices (Neuromonics, etc.). In addition, the clinicians questioned whether the presentation of loud

sounds during testing triggered the seizure event. We recommended the use of sound therapy utilizing a sleep band headband, which is soft and fits loosely over the ears and head. LO felt that this was a viable option. We also carefully explained the testing results, the recommendations, and the use of sound therapy to her friend in case LO had been distracted during counseling due to the seizure activity. In addition, we gave LO some desensitization exercises to help her manage her hyperacusis symptoms. We encouraged meeting with her medical doctors and discussing the outcomes of the tinnitus and sound sensitivity evaluation.

2.7 Outcome

LO met with her neurologist and pain management doctors a few weeks after our visit. She indicated that her neurologist was "more concerned with the seizures" at that point than the tinnitus management. Her pain management doctor, however, was familiar with the desensitization exercises that she had been given by our clinic and highly encouraged her to continue with the protocol. He also put together a list of things for her to try to improve her quality of life, particularly with her migraines and neck pain, including pool and physical therapies. She also received Botox injections for her migraines.

2.8 Self-Efficacy Considerations for the Clinician

- Tinnitus and hyperacusis management options can be modified based on a patient's case history and touch/sensation sensitivity to include delivery of desensitization stimuli with a headband rather than ear-level maskers.
- Tinnitus symptoms may worsen over time and follow-up appointments and additional therapy options will need to be explored, including amplification, tinnitus maskers, or standalone sound therapy devices.
- Tinnitus and sound sensitivity treatment can easily incorporate a team management approach, including audiologists, physicians, psychologists and related mental health professionals, physical and occupational therapists, and others. Clinicians should make every effort to communicate with a patient's other health care providers, especially in cases of complicated medical histories. Information sharing is a must.

References

[1] Newman CW, Jacobson GP, Spitzer JB. Development of the Tinnitus Handicap Inventory. Arch Otolaryngol Head Neck Surg. 1996; 122(2):143–148

[2] Meikle MB, Henry JA, Griest SE, et al. The tinnitus functional index: development of a new clinical measure for chronic, intrusive tinnitus. Ear Hear. 2012; 33(2):153–176

[3] Eggermont J. Animal models of hyperacusis and decreased sound tolerance in Fagelson and Baguley hyperacusis and disorders of sound tolerance: clinical and research perspectives. San Diego, CA: Plural Publishing; 2018

[4] Paulin J, Andersson L, Nordin S. Characteristics of hyperacusis in the general population. Noise Health. 2016; 18(83):178–184

[5] McFerran D. Hyperacusis: medical diagnosis and associated syndromes in Fagelson and Baguley hyperacusis and disorders of sound tolerance: clinical and research perspectives. San Diego, CA: Plural Publishing; 2018

[6] Jastreboff PJ, Jastreboff MM. Treatments for decreased sound tolerance (hyperacusis and misophonia). In: Seminars in hearing, Vol. 35. New York: Thieme Medical Publishers; 2014:105–120

Suggested Reading

Mancarella C, Delfini R, Landi A. Chiari malformations. Acta Neurochirurgica 2019;125:89–95

3 Tinnitus Treatment Following Acoustic Neuroma and Meniere's Disease: A Single Case Study

Ann Perreau and Richard S. Tyler

3.1 Clinical History

This case involves a 60-year-old female with chronic, bilateral sensorineural tinnitus following right-sided acoustic neuroma removal by an otologist. The patient's hearing could not be preserved after tumor removal, resulting in profound deafness in the right ear. The patient had mild-to-moderate sensorineural hearing loss in the left ear and was fit with a Bi-CROS hearing aid by her local audiologist. At that time, her tinnitus was manageable and the hearing aid was helpful in improving communication abilities at work and at home. However, about 1.6 years after acoustic neuroma removal, the patient experienced a dramatic increase in her tinnitus in the left ear that was distressing and debilitating. She described the tinnitus as both a siren and whooshing sound that lasted for 2 weeks. Because of the increased tinnitus, the patient returned to her otologist for a consultation. Based on her symptoms of left sensorineural hearing loss, fluctuating tinnitus, and no vertigo, the otologist diagnosed her with cochlear Meniere's disease in the left ear. This diagnosis was subsequently confirmed by two outside otologists. She was referred to the Augustana College Center for Speech, Language, and Hearing for management of her tinnitus.

3.2 Audiologic Testing

Pure-tone audiometry was consistent with profound sensorineural hearing loss in the right ear and a moderate low-frequency sensorineural hearing loss in the left ear. The patient's audiogram is presented in ▶ Fig. 3.1. The patient reported no history of ear infections, no vertigo or dizziness, and no history of noise exposure. There was a family history of hearing loss due to aging. Health history revealed no other chronic or serious illnesses, except for medications for high blood pressure and seasonal allergies.

3.3 Questions for the Reader

1. Is severe tinnitus a possible complication following acoustic neuroma surgery?
2. Should an audiologist consider fitting a contralateral routing of signal (CROS) hearing aid system for patients with unilateral deafness following tumor removal?
3. Do all patients with Meniere's disease report vertigo as a symptom?

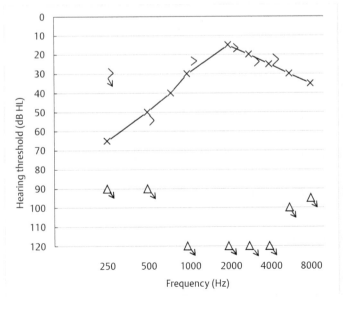

Fig. 3.1 Patient's audiogram showing right and left ear hearing thresholds for frequencies 250–8000 Hz.

3.4 Discussion of Questions for the Reader

1. *Is severe tinnitus a possible complication following acoustic neuroma surgery?*
   Yes, tinnitus is a possible complication following surgical removal of an acoustic neuroma, occurring in less than 10% of cases.[1] However, tinnitus more commonly occurs preoperatively for patients who are diagnosed with an acoustic neuroma (73% of cases) and can be the presenting complaint in about 11% of cases.[2]
2. *Should an audiologist consider fitting a contralateral routing of signal hearing aid (i.e., CROS, Bi-CROS) for patients with unilateral deafness following tumor removal?*
   Yes, a trial with CROS devices is recommended for patients who have hearing loss as a result of tumor removal. The evidence on the effectiveness of CROS devices for tinnitus reduction or suppression in this population is lacking, although studies have shown positive results on speech recognition tests when using CROS devices.[1]
3. *Do all patients with Meniere's disease report vertigo as a symptom?*
   No, not all patients with Meniere's disease will report vertigo as a symptom. Cochlear Meniere's disease is diagnosed when a patient presents with auditory symptoms of Meniere's disease (i.e., hearing loss, aural fullness, and roaring tinnitus), but no vestibular symptoms (i.e., vertigo). Cochlear Meniere's disease likely represents endolymphatic hydrops of the cochlear duct.

3.5 Additional Testing

Beyond audiometric testing, several questionnaires were administered to document the patient's hearing history (our clinic's hearing intake questionnaire), spatial hearing ability (Spatial Hearing Questionnaire[3]—short version), and tinnitus severity (Tinnitus Handicap Questionnaire[4] or THQ). In addition, the 12-item Tinnitus Primary Functions Questionnaire[5] (TPFQ) was administered to determine her reactions to tinnitus. Questionnaire results shown in ▶ Table 3.1 suggested that her tinnitus was bothersome, and that her thoughts and emotions and hearing abilities were influenced substantially by her tinnitus. We then identified three goals for therapy using the Client Oriented Scale of Improvement in Tinnitus[6] (COSIT) which is based on

Table 3.1 Results from three questionnaires: SHQ-S, THQ, and TPFQ administered to the patient

Questionnaire (total score/ subscale)	Patient score (range among items)
1. SHQ-S	
SHQ-S Total score	16.7 (0–50)
Speech in spatially separated noise subscale	50.0 (50)
Sound Localization subscale	0.0 (0)
2. THQ	
THQ Total score	40.7 (0–100)
Social, emotional, and physical subscale	30.7 (0–50)
Hearing subscale	64.2 (30–100)
3. TPFQ	
TPFQ Total score	48.8 (20–80)
Concentration subscale	28.3 (25–30)
Emotion subscale	78.3 (60–80)
Hearing subscale	53.3 (30–80)
Sleep subscale	40.0 (20–50)

Abbreviations: SHQ-S, Spatial Hearing Questionnaire-Short; THQ, Tinnitus Handicap Questionnaire; TPFQ, Tinnitus Primary Functions Questionnaire.
Note: All questionnaires are scored 0–100. Higher scores on SHQ-S indicate better spatial hearing ability, whereas higher scores on the THQ and TPFQ indicate greater tinnitus severity or worse reactions to tinnitus.

the modified Client Oriented Scale of Improvement[7] (COSI). We specifically targeted: (a) her fears that she would become deaf and her tinnitus would get worse, (b) her avoidance of noisy situations such as church and restaurants with family, and (c) her anxiety about tinnitus interfering with daily activities such as work.

3.6 Final Diagnosis and Recommended Treatment

The patient approached our clinic for tinnitus management, and she received both group and individual counseling. At the initial tinnitus group educational session, we educated the patient about tinnitus, hearing, hearing loss, and attention, and reviewed treatment options. She met others with tinnitus, discussed her experiences with tinnitus as it relates to others, and learned that she was not alone.

In our individual counseling sessions, we addressed the patient's negative thought patterns

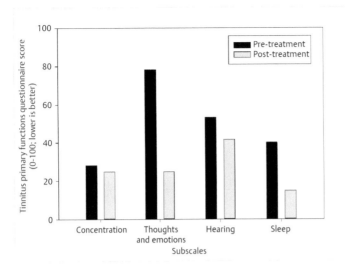

Fig. 3.2 Pre- and posttreatment results from Tinnitus Primary Functions Questionnaire for the four subscales.

related to tinnitus and demonstrated communication strategies and relaxation techniques to improve hearing and sleep, respectively. Specifically, we used the Tinnitus Activities Treatment[8]: Introduction and Thoughts and Emotions sessions to explore how tinnitus has influenced her life, and how one attends to auditory stimuli. In addition, the counseling considered how thoughts dictate emotions, how one can modify negative thought patterns related to tinnitus and, as a result, can improve the ability to manage the effects of tinnitus. We also discussed her hearing loss and appropriate sound therapy options to decrease the prominence of her tinnitus. Because the patient has unilateral hearing loss, we emphasized the importance of using low-level stimuli to minimize interference with speech understanding. When her tinnitus increased associated with Meniere's disease, the patient began using masking sounds through her Bi-CROS hearing aid up to 12 h/d. She listened to low-level music, which was relaxing to her and preferred it to nature sounds for low-level background sound.

Finally, the patient kept a diary of her thoughts and emotions as they related to tinnitus, logging activities, and sounds that affected tinnitus to determine the next steps in her journey toward acceptance. The diary revealed that her tinnitus was more bothersome at night than during the day; therefore, the sleep session of Tinnitus Activities Treatment was also reviewed. The patient was aware of many things that affected her sleep, including caffeine intake, and ways to promote better sleep using low-level background sound, including a fan and white noise from her tablet.

3.7 Outcomes

After 2 months of counseling using Tinnitus Activities Treatment, the patient's TPFQ scores revealed a significant improvement in her reactions to tinnitus for several subscales (refer to ▶ Fig. 3.2), especially for thoughts and emotions and sleep.

After therapy, using the COSIT to document treatment effectiveness, the patient reported that her hearing difficulties were reduced, avoidance of social situations was slightly better (still prefers to avoid noisy places), and her enjoyment of daily life was much improved. Although her tinnitus fluctuates from time to time, she reports that she now enjoys work and social activities with less fear and anxiety about her tinnitus. Specifically, her reactions to the fluctuating loudness of her tinnitus are improved because she has implemented many of the approaches from therapy into her daily life.

Acknowledgment

Thanks to our tinnitus patients for providing the inspiration for this case study and our work.

References

[1] Baguley DM, Williamson CA, Moffat DA. Treating tinnitus in patients with otologic conditions. In: Tyler RS, ed. Tinnitus treatment: clinical protocols. New York: Thieme; 2006:41–50

[2] Moffat DA, Baguley DM, Beynon GJ, Da Cruz M. Clinical acumen and vestibular schwannoma. Am J Otol. 1998; 19(1): 82–87

[3] Ou H, Perreau A, Tyler RS. Development of a shortened version of the Spatial Hearing Questionnaire (SHQ-S) for screening spatial-hearing ability. Am J Audiol. 2017; 26(3):293–300

[4] Kuk FK, Tyler RS, Russell D, Jordan H. The psychometric properties of a tinnitus handicap questionnaire. Ear Hear. 1990; 11(6):434–445

[5] Tyler R, Ji H, Perreau A, Witt S, Noble W, Coelho C. Development and validation of the tinnitus primary function questionnaire. Am J Audiol. 2014; 23(3):260–272

[6] Searchfield GD. A Client Oriented Scale of Improvement in tinnitus for therapy goal planning and assessing outcomes. J Am Acad Audiol. 2019; 30:327-337. DOI: https://doi.org/10.3766/jaaa.17119

[7] Dillon H, James A, Ginis J. Client Oriented Scale of Improvement (COSI) and its relationship to several other measures of benefit and satisfaction provided by hearing aids. J Am Acad Audiol. 1997; 8(1):27–43

[8] Tyler RS, Gehringer AK, Noble W, Dunn CC, Witt SA, Bardia A. Tinnitus activities treatment. In: Tyler RS, ed. Tinnitus treatment: clinical protocols. New York: Thieme; 2006: 116–132

Suggested Reading

Tyler RS, Haskell GB, Gogel SA, Gehringer AK. Establishing a tinnitus clinic in your practice. Am J Audiol. 2008; 17(1):25–37

Tyler RS, Noble W, Coelho C, Roncancio E, Jun HJ. Tinnitus and hyperacusis. In: Katz J, Chasin M, English K, Hood L, Tillery K, eds. Handbook of clinical audiology. 7th ed. Baltimore, MD: Lippincott Williams & Wilkins; 2015:647–658

4 A Case of Pulsatile Tinnitus with Predictable Pattern of Occurrence

Catherine M. Edmonds

4.1 Clinical History/Description

An 80-year-old male patient was seen at the audiology clinic in 2013 reporting pulsatile tinnitus in the left ear and difficulty hearing in both ears, worse in the right ear. The patient also reported he could not hear on the telephone in the right ear, but he could with the left ear. He stated that he was receiving ENT care at a different facility for unilateral (left) pulsatile tinnitus and reportedly had a computed tomography (CT) scan showing "mastoid opacification." In addition, he stated he was seeking a secondary ENT opinion at another facility for treatment of the tinnitus and was interested in receiving "mastoid surgery" was not recommended by the first consulting ENT physician. He reported the tinnitus commenced in 2012 in the left ear and related it to "possibly happening after a left ear flushing" or a fall in 2012 when he struck his head. The nature of the tinnitus was described by the patient as the sound of his pulse accompanied by a ringing, buzzing sound that he heard for 3 days and 3 nights then stopped completely for 2 days and 2 nights. He reiterated, "I hear my pulse" during these episodes; however, he did not describe the tinnitus as increasing in rate with his pulse, such as during physical exertion. The patient also reported the tinnitus consistently began in the middle of the night when "lying flat" at which times he stated that it woke him up. In addition, he reported "dripping of fluid" from his nose each time the tinnitus occurred, resolving when the tinnitus ceased. Audiologic history was positive for bilateral, asymmetric sensorineural hearing loss, but negative for ear surgery, otalgia, tympanic membrane (TM) perforation, dizziness, vertigo, facial numbness or tingling, sound intolerance, conductive or mixed hearing loss, and hearing aid use. He did not provide previous medical records.

4.2 Audiologic Testing

Audiometric testing revealed asymmetric sensorineural hearing loss (SNHL) with poorer results for the right ear (non-tinnitus ear). Word recognition scores were asymmetric, also poorer in the right (non-tinnitus) ear using W-22 and NU-6 recorded stimuli. Tympanometry indicated a type C tympanogram left and a type A tympanogram right (▶ Fig. 4.1). Acoustic stapedial reflex thresholds could not be obtained as the clinician could not sustain an airtight seal in either ear. Referral for otologic management of pulsatile tinnitus was required per clinic policy. The patient was referred to neurotologist as he had already consulted an ENT physician with second ENT opinion pending.

4.3 Questions for the Reader

1. Why should a report of pulsatile tinnitus be referred for otologic evaluation?
2. Why might a report of fluid leak from the nose concurrent with pulsatile tinnitus be of importance to the diagnosis of this patient?
3. What audiologic services should be offered to support this particular case of pulsatile tinnitus and hearing loss?

4.4 Discussion of Questions for the Reader

1. *Why should a report of pulsatile tinnitus be referred for otologic evaluation?*
   Diagnosis of pulsatile tinnitus requires physical examination and imaging studies in order to rule out vascular disorder and/or the presence of a potentially dangerous arterial-venous malformation (AVM). Such examinations are outside the scope of audiologic practice. Treatment is dependent on the source of the pulsatile tinnitus, but may involve surgical intervention, also outside the scope of audiologic practice.[1]
2. *Why might a report of fluid leak from the nose concurrent with pulsatile tinnitus be of importance to the diagnosis of this patient?*
   Fluid running from the nose concurrent with pulsatile tinnitus is suspicious for cerebrospinal fluid (CSF) leak and supports the rationale for otologic physical examination and imaging studies for diagnosis.[2]
3. *What audiologic services should be offered to support this particular case of pulsatile tinnitus and hearing loss?*
   Combination of hearing aids/tinnitus sound-generating devices programmed to real ear

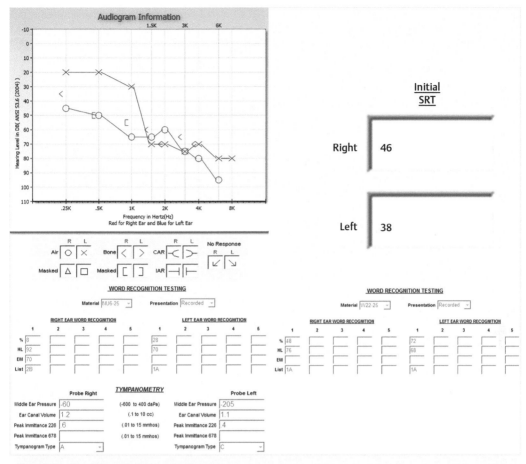

Fig. 4.1 Results of the audiologic evaluation.

targets and assistive listening devices as needed due to the poor word recognition ability should be provided. Evidence-based tinnitus services including counseling with audiology and mental health providers and bedside or environmental sound-generating devices are within the audiologists' scope. Outcome measures for both hearing aids and tinnitus as well as ongoing follow-up support for hearing and tinnitus needs based on the patient's request for care should also be provided. Audiology should continue to coordinate care with otology in the event of change in current symptoms or if new symptoms arise.[3]

4.5 Additional Testing

Magnetic resonance imaging (MRI) of the head with attention to the internal auditory canals (IAC)

and CT scan was ultimately ordered by a neurotologist. The MRI demonstrated no mass of the IAC, inner ear, or cerebellopontine angle. There was fluid within the left mastoid with a similar hyperintensity to CSF on T2 imaging. On CT scan, there was also opacification within the mastoid. The tegmen was very thin, especially the tegmen tympani. A thin layer of bone not consistent with canal dehiscence, covered the superior semicircular canal. There was no sigmoid sinus diverticulum. There was no mass of the middle ear or jugular foramen.

4.6 Final Diagnosis and Recommended Treatment

Spontaneous CSF leak into the left mastoid was confirmed; surgical intervention was not recommended by the consulting neurotologist based on risk of hearing loss to the better hearing ear, and risk of postoperative complication to the better hearing ear, and patient's health issues. CI candidacy was not likely due to complicating health factors should hearing loss result from surgical intervention; recall from the history, the patient reportedly could only hear on the telephone with the left ear. Patient was advised by the neurotologist to continue to receive Pneumovax vaccination every 5 years and to seek otologic follow-up if changes or new symptoms occurred. Treatment provided included hearing instruments with active tinnitus sound generator, television assistive listening device (ALD) paired to the hearing instruments, completion of Progressive Tinnitus Management (PTM) workshops with audiology and mental health support incorporated into the sessions, continued use of PTM skills including use of therapeutic sound and elements of cognitive behavior therapy (CBT) skills when tinnitus was present and bothersome. Bedside sound generator for sleep disturbance due to tinnitus as needed was provided for the patient.

4.7 Outcomes

Last contact with the patient in 2016 indicated continued left pulsatile tinnitus occurring in the aforementioned pattern of 2 to 3 days of bothersome tinnitus followed by 2 to 3 days with no tinnitus. The patient remained an inconsistent hearing instrument user in spite of his report, while in the clinic he "could barely hear" his tinnitus when wearing his hearing aids. He admittedly used his bedside sound conditioner infrequently and reported that he was taking Clonazepam for sleep disturbance related to the tinnitus prescribed by a private primary care physician. He returned to the neurotologist to request surgical intervention in the left ear regardless of the risks but was denied by the neurotologist whose medical opinion was that the risks outweighed the potential benefits due to the complicated nature of the surgical procedure and the patients' other health issues. The patient reported that the additional ENT physicians he consulted also declined to render surgical intervention.

References

[1] Kleinjung T. Pulsatile tinnitus. In: Baguley DM, Fagelson M, eds. Tinnitus clinical and research perspectives. San Diego, CA: Plural Publishing; 2016:163–180

[2] Pelosi S, Bederson JB, Smouha EE. Cerebrospinal fluid leaks of temporal bone origin: selection of surgical approach. Skull Base. 2010; 20(4):253–259

[3] Adult tinnitus management clinical practice. https://www.ncrar.research.va.gov/Documents/TinnitusPracticeGuidelines.pdf

Suggested Readings

Baguley DM, Fagelson M. Pulsatile tinnitus. In: Tinnitus clinical and research perspectives. San Diego, CA: Plural Publishing; 2016:163–180

AAO HNS Clinical Practice Guideline: Tinnitus Otolaryngology–Head and Neck Surgery 2014, Vol. 151(2S) S1–S40 © American Academy of Otolaryngology—Head and Neck Surgery Foundation 2014 Reprints and permission: sagepub.com/journalsPermissions.nav DOI: 10.1177/0194599814545325 http://otojournal.org

National Center for Rehabilitative Auditory Research: Progressive Tinnitus Management https://www.ncrar.research.va.gov/Clinician Resources/IndexPTM.asp

Pelosi S, Bederson JB, Smouha EE. Cerebrospinal fluid leaks of temporal bone origin: selection of surgical approach. Skull Base. 2010;20(4):253-259. doi:10.1055/s-0030-1249249

Disclaimer

5 Otosclerosis with Tinnitus

Lauren Mann

5.1 Clinical History and Presentation

CA is an 81-year-old male reporting recurrent bothersome tinnitus for 2 years. He was seen 2 years ago by a hearing instrument specialist complaining of tinnitus and was given a standard pure-tone air and bone conduction test. He presented with bilateral severe presbycusis with additional severe, low-frequency asymmetric conductive hearing loss, which was worse in the right ear. CA was not referred to a physician at that point. Instead, he was given a medical waiver and encouraged to pursue amplification for the hearing loss and tinnitus. CA spent roughly $4,000 on bilateral receiver-in-the-canal (RIC) devices and wore them for 6 months. At that point, he was still experiencing the same discomfort with tinnitus and did not feel his hearing had improved at all. He scheduled testing with an audiologist at an otolaryngology practice and he was ultimately diagnosed with otosclerosis. A stapedectomy and prosthetic implant subsequently produced a partial recovery of low-frequency hearing, leaving a mild-to-severe sensorineural loss at 4,000 Hz and above. CA continued to experience bothersome tinnitus one year following his surgery, and he was therefore referred to our clinic for an evaluation.

Our clinical protocol is based on the NCRAR Progressive Tinnitus Management (PTM) program[1] and the Jastreboff model of tinnitus retraining therapy (TRT) for sound therapy administration.[2] Following audiometric testing and appropriate trial with amplification, we move to pitch and loudness assessment and determination of candidacy for sound therapy or additional supports. At all levels of interaction, patients are provided with a 30-minute counseling session. This session includes specific instruction on biofeedback exercises such as progressive muscle relaxation (PMR) or diaphragmatic breathing (DB). Patients are asked to complete 1 to 3 minutes of exercises when unable to ignore tinnitus and return to activity.

In our clinic, CA reported good general health with comorbid hypertension and hypothyroidism; both of which were being pharmacologically managed. He reported parental history of hearing loss; denied significant noise exposure, head injury, dizziness, and fullness in the ears. He reported sensitivity to loud sounds and indicated difficulty hearing in background noise. His Tinnitus Handicap Inventory (THI)[3] score of 56 indicated a moderate degree of tinnitus impairment and he reported hearing it mostly in the right ear. He completed a Characteristics of Amplification Tool (COAT) questionnaire[4] indicating minimal concern with hearing loss and he subjectively rated hearing ability as a 7/10.

5.2 Audiological Evaluation

Otoscopy indicated clear, patent canals and normal eardrum appearance on the left side but an opaque eardrum on the right, consistent with surgical history. Pure-tone air and bone conduction testing revealed a mild-to-moderate sensorineural hearing loss at 3,000 Hz and above in the left ear. Right ear thresholds revealed an asymmetric mild-to-severe mixed hearing loss consistent with the previous audiogram obtained at the otolaryngology office. The Loudness Contour Test[5] indicated a reduced tolerance for pure tones in both ears with thresholds of discomfort between 80 and 90 dB HL. Speech testing is not standard in all tinnitus appointments but was included per the patient's concern that his ability to hear his family had diminished after he quit hearing aid use. His speech recognition thresholds (SRT) were consistent with the pure-tone average (PTA) and word recognition scores were both 100% at 40 dB SL regarding the 2,000-Hz threshold with contralateral masking (▶ Fig. 5.1).

Tympanometry was normal for the left ear (Jerger Type A) and showed reduced compliance for the right (Jerger Type A_s), consistent with surgical history. Acoustic reflex thresholds (ARTs) were not assessed for pure tones due to patient discomfort. Our clinical protocol includes a test of loudness tolerance at pure-tone ART frequencies and ART testing is not conducted if the test levels would exceed the patient's tolerance. Broadband noise ARTs were present at expected levels for the probe-left conditions and absent for probe-right conditions (▶ Fig. 5.2).

Tinnitus pitch and loudness assessment matched CA's tinnitus to a pure tone of 4,000 Hz at 13 dB SL with reference stimuli played in the left ear. CA's minimum masking level (MML) was 26 dB SL (44 dB HL) using white noise. He experienced

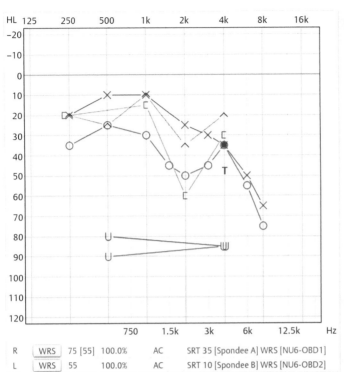

Fig. 5.1 Audiogram.

R	WRS	75 [55]	100.0%	AC	SRT 35 [Spondee A] WRS [NU6-OBD1]
L	WRS	55	100.0%	AC	SRT 10 [Spondee B] WRS [NU6-OBD2]

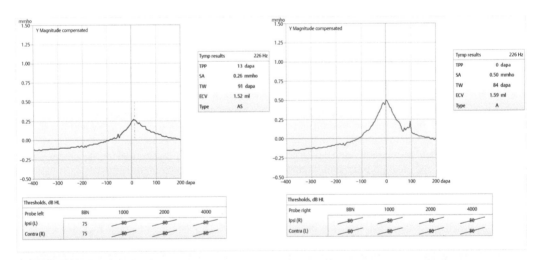

Fig. 5.2 Immitance.

32 seconds of residual inhibition (RI) following a one-minute masker presentation at 54 dB HL. Following RI testing, CA reported his tinnitus was significantly lower in perceived volume. By the end of the appointment, he reported that the volume had not returned to normal levels indicating a maintained partial inhibition of symptoms (▶ Fig. 5.3).

After testing, CA was given a Tinnitus Functional Index (TFI) questionnaire[6] to help determine the appropriate sound therapy route. Levo System candidacy includes a TFI score of 25 or higher.[7] He scored a 51 indicating he was a candidate for the Levo system overnight intervention or a hearing aid with sound therapy available for waking hours.

Tinnitus Evaluation	Stimulus Ear		
	Right	Binaural	Left
Pitch Matching			T 4000 Hz
Loudness Matching			T 13 SL
Hearing Threshold			● 35 HL
Masking Noise Threshold	18 HL	18 HL	6 HL
Minimum Masking Level (MML)	26 SL (44 HL)		
Maskability	Complete		
Residual Inhibition	32 s		
Inhibition Characteristic	Complete		

Note: Reduced gain post-RI

Fig. 5.3 Tinnitus evaluation.

5.3 Questions for the Reader

1. Do you think CA is a good candidate for amplification? For sound therapy?
2. Is tinnitus a common symptom of otosclerosis?
3. How would you address the dispenser's negligence in not appropriately referring CA for the conductive asymmetry?
4. What additional tinnitus strategies might be appropriate in this case?

5.4 Discussion of Questions for the Reader

1. *Do you think CA is a good candidate for amplification? For sound therapy?*
   In the right ear, CA has thresholds all within the mild-to-moderate range through 6,000 Hz. His left ear has normal hearing through 2,000 Hz; however, he did present with sound sensitivity. CA did not report complaints of hearing loss, other than those noted in small groups of family. He presented with a history of surgical intervention for otosclerosis, so we could be confident his thresholds would not improve further with medical intervention. For these reasons, we recommended bilateral amplification for the management of tinnitus and sound sensitivity.
2. *Is tinnitus a common symptom of otosclerosis?*
   Although not a common symptom, there is significant evidence that patients may experience tinnitus due to the middle ear and possible secondary inner ear dysfunction produced by stapes fixation. There are reports of improved tinnitus following surgical intervention, but this was not the case for this patient. (See Deggouj et al[8] for a review.)
3. *How would you address the dispenser's negligence in not appropriately referring CA for the conductive asymmetry?*
   The dispenser had CA sign a medical waiver to proceed with amplification, but CA did not remember signing it or discussing any reason to seek a physician's care. He found the document later. Unfortunately, CA was past the 30-day trial period by the time he saw an audiologist at an otolaryngology practice, so he ultimately had to keep the devices and felt as though he had no recourse. The hearing aids were private-labeled and not open for programming by other offices, so when referred to our clinic for tinnitus, we were unable to use the current amplification as an option. We proceeded with a new device in our practice that would allow for amplification and sound therapy. The patient asked for assistance in filing a complaint with the state dispensing license office and we provided CA with contact information to do so. He filed a report outlining the lack of appropriate referral, given his asymmetrical conductive hearing loss and unilateral tinnitus. He reported not being fully informed on the nature of his hearing loss nor appropriate management for tinnitus, which was his primary complaint.
4. *What additional tinnitus strategies might be appropriate in this case?*
   Following a progressive management strategy, CA would move on toward team-based care if

he did not improve with amplification and sound therapy. We considered a nighttime sound therapy (LEVO) option for CA but given his additional hearing loss and complaints of tinnitus during waking hours, it was determined that daytime sound therapy would be the best initial plan. Our team-based care progresses to cognitive behavioral therapy (CBT), psychology, psychiatry, sleep clinic, and/or neurology depending on severity and comorbid symptoms.

5.5 Recommendations and Outcomes

Given CA's MML, we could safely set a mixing point for TRT below 50 dBSPL and CA was set up with RIC devices to provide mild amplification and TRT. Since return to sleep was a significant complaint, we instructed CA to use an app-based masker in his room overnight to avoid waking into complete quiet. CA's 1-month follow-up THI score was 42 and TFI was 36. CA's Client-Oriented Scale of Improvement (COSI) questionnaire[9] suggested he was pleased with the reduction in duration and loudness of his tinnitus. CA additionally reported hearing better in small groups and was better tolerating the collective sound level in groups. His 3-month follow-up THI score was 28 and TFI was 30. CA reported tinnitus being at a manageable level and he was not interested in pursuing CBT or additional strategies for tinnitus or sound sensitivity management. He was successfully practicing PMR to assist with sleep, and he reported moving from a full-body circuit to barely making it through one arm before falling asleep. He attributes much of his improvement in tinnitus to his improved sleep.

5.6 Key Points

- Hearing aid dispensers often fill an important need in the diagnosis and management of hearing loss; however, it is imperative that any provider prescribing amplification make appropriate medical referrals. Without appropriate referral, patients may spend a significant amount of time, money, and distress before receiving the care they need. Audiologists can and should offer to be a resource for local dispensers when atypical hearing losses or symptom presentations occur.
- Although there is no cure for tinnitus, appropriate treatment may result in a significant reduction in tinnitus perception and impact. It is important to use a variety of outcome assessments to determine if a patient is coping with their tinnitus or requires additional referrals for care.

References

[1] Henry J. Progressive tinnitus management: clinical handbook for audiologists. Plural Pub.; 2010
[2] Jastreboff PJ, Jastreboff MM. Tinnitus Retraining Therapy (TRT) as a method for treatment of tinnitus and hyperacusis patients. J Am Acad Audiol. 2000; 11(3):162–177
[3] Newman CW, Jacobson GP, Spitzer JB. Development of the Tinnitus Handicap Inventory. Arch Otolaryngol Head Neck Surg. 1996; 122(2):143–148
[4] Sandridge S, Newman C. (2006) Improving the efficiency and accountability of the hearing aid selection process—use of the COAT. Audiology online accessed on December 1st 2020
[5] Cox RM, Alexander GC, Taylor IM, Gray GA. The contour test of loudness perception. Ear Hear. 1997; 18(5):388–400
[6] Meikle MB, Henry JA, Griest SE, et al. The tinnitus functional index: development of a new clinical measure for chronic, intrusive tinnitus. Ear Hear. 2012; 33(2):153–176
[7] Theodoroff SM, McMillan GP, Zaugg TL, Cheslock M, Roberts C, Henry JA. Randomized controlled trial of a novel device for tinnitus sound therapy during sleep. Am J Audiol. 2017; 26 (4):543–554
[8] Deggouj N, Castelein S, Gerard JM, Decat M, Gersdorff M. Tinnitus and otosclerosis. B-ENT. 2009; 5(4):241–244
[9] Dillon H, James A, Ginis J. Client Oriented Scale of Improvement (COSI) and its relationship to several other measures of benefit and satisfaction provided by hearing aids. J Am Acad Audiol. 1997; 8(1):27–43

6 Tinnitus Following Concussion

Lauren Mann

6.1 Clinical History and Presentation

DD is a 40-year-old female seen for sudden-onset tinnitus following a recent motor-vehicle accident. She was rear-ended and sustained a whiplash injury and occipital lobe impact. She was seen by our concussion interdisciplinary team 7 months later as symptoms persisted. At intake, her Post Concussion Symptom Scale[15] score of 77 included vision loss, imbalance when walking, sound sensitivity, significant sleep disturbance, a central tremor, and anxiety. This inventory does not include tinnitus; however, DD reported tinnitus complaints to the neurologists, specifically in her left ear.

During her tinnitus evaluation, the initial Tinnitus Handicap Inventory (THI[17]) score was 68 (severe), Tinnitus Functional Index (TFI[16]) was 76 (severe), and Beck Depression Screening PC[4] score of 7 was normal. She reported no family history or complaints of hearing loss, no significant noise exposure, and no previous history of otologic disorders or surgery. Her medication list did not include any known sources of tinnitus. She reported tinnitus in the left ear at the time of evaluation and indicated the most disturbance during the day; she did not report difficulty falling asleep due to tinnitus. She attributed her reported sleep disturbance (as reported to neurology) to significant anxiety.

6.2 Audiological Evaluation

DD's pure-tone air and bone conduction testing was conducted with the booth door ajar per her request and revealed an asymmetric loss. DD had normal hearing through 6,000 Hz in the right ear with mild-to-moderate sensorineural hearing loss (SNHL) at 8,000 Hz and above, while her left ear's thresholds revealed mild-to-moderate SNHL above 3,000 Hz (▸ Fig. 6.1).

Immittance testing indicated Jerger Type A tympanograms bilaterally. Acoustic reflex thresholds (ART) were not conducted due to uncomfortable loudness (UCL) levels, which had been obtained at 80 to 90 dB HL for each ear when presented with pure tones at ART frequencies. ART testing at 80 dB was initiated at 1 kHz and using BBN but aborted due to discomfort reported (▸ Fig. 6.2).

Distortion product otoacoustic emissions (DPOAE) were present at a 6-dB signal-to-noise ratio (SNR) and found at normal amplitudes for 8/13 test frequencies from 750 to 8,000 Hz in the right compared to 4/13 test frequencies in the left (▸ Fig. 6.3).

Tinnitus pitch was matched to 9,000 Hz at 12 dB sensation level (dB SL) with reference stimulus played in the right ear and DD comparing our stimuli to her left. Subsequent presentations in the left ear confirmed the pitch was perceived as similar to her tinnitus. DD became upset during pitch and loudness testing; she was concerned she was not performing well on the test. DD indicated it was extremely important to her that we know her precise tinnitus pitch. We stopped testing for a break and counseled on the testing and management process. It was important that DD understand that our testing approximated tinnitus and was used to better diagnose her tinnitus symptoms and to help us determine the treatment options available for her. In other words, her collective test results helped us determine what might be beneficial for her. Once returning to testing, minimum masking level (MML) was found at 58 dB SL with white noise in the left ear and 46 dB SL in the binaural condition. Due to the high dB HL required for MML in the left condition, residual inhibition testing was completed in the binaural condition only and she experienced 3 seconds of inhibition following a 1-minute white noise presentation. Once the tinnitus returned, she reported no changes in perceived pitch or volume compared to initial tinnitus. DD requested to drive the testing herself, so we proceeded to have DD self-match her tinnitus using the Levo Tinnitus Manager. She localized her tinnitus at 8,558 Hz and we noted that the process took DD 15 minutes to complete. She repeatedly started the sound over and took four trials to feel confident she had found the correct pitch and loudness. DD felt significantly reassured when we discussed results and her Levo-match was close to the pitch found during our testing (▸ Fig. 6.4).

6.3 Questions for the Reader

1. Do you think DD is a good candidate for amplification? For sound therapy?

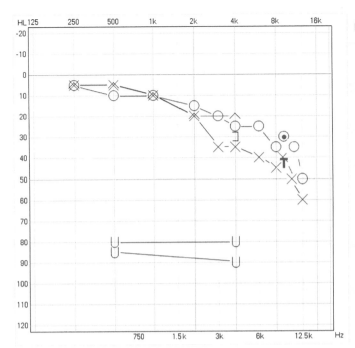

Fig. 6.1 Audiogram.

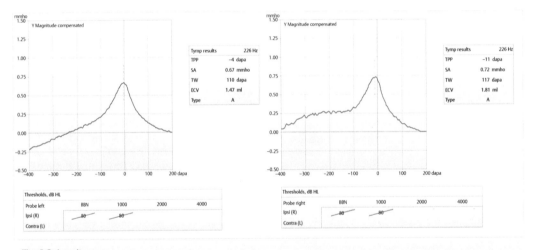

Fig. 6.2 Immitance.

2. Is tinnitus a common symptom of concussion?
3. Are sleep recommendations within the scope of practice for audiologists?
4. Would the inclusion of ARTs add diagnostic value to this assessment?
5. If a patient is managing their tinnitus well with Tinnitus Retraining Therapy (TRT), should they continue using it indefinitely?

6.4 Discussion of Questions for the Reader

1. *Do you think DD is a good candidate for amplification? For sound therapy?*
   DD has a mild hearing loss at 6000 Hz and above in the right ear, indicating little room to benefit from amplification. The left ear showed

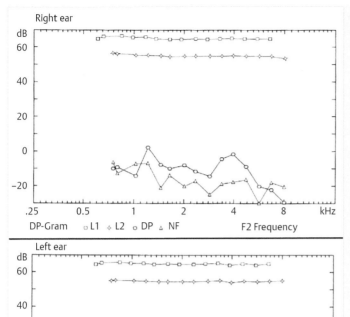

Fig. 6.3 Distortion product otoacoustic emissions (DPOAEs).

Tinnitus Evaluation	Stimulus Ear		
	Right	**Binaural**	**Left**
Pitch Matching	T 9000 Hz		T 9000 Hz
Loudness Matching	T 12 SL		
Hearing Threshold	● 30 HL		
Masking Noise Threshold	-4 HL	-10 HL	-2 HL
Minimum Masking Level (MML)		46 SL (36 HL)	58 SL (56 HL)
Maskability		Complete	Complete
Residual Inhibition		3 s	
Inhibition Characteristic		Complete	
Note: no change post RI			

Fig. 6.4 Tinnitus evaluation.

mild-to-moderate hearing loss starting at 3,000 Hz, which would be expected to exert some influence on communication. However, she did not report a hearing loss nor indicate any hearing difficulties during intake. Although DD was adamantly against hearing aids, we felt recommending amplification was important in this instance, to address DD's tinnitus, hearing loss, and co-occurring anxiety. We were careful to counsel on the purpose of amplification for tinnitus treatment and as a method of auditory enrichment, in addition to benefits she might experience with communication.

2. *Is tinnitus a common symptom of concussion?*
   Tinnitus is a known symptom of concussion but reports of incidence vary greatly: 0 to 62.5% across populations.[5,6,7,8,10,14,18,19,21,22] It is difficult to understand the true effects of head injury on the auditory system when much of the current literature involves military populations with comorbid noise exposure. Importantly, sudden-onset tinnitus following a head injury and whiplash often produces a much higher mental burden for the patient, compared to nontrauma-induced tinnitus.[9,13]

3. *Are sleep recommendations within the scope of practice for audiologists?*
   It is commonly held that chronic tinnitus and sleep disturbance are related.[2] Assessing sleep quality using case questions or validated questionnaires and providing recommendations to improve sleep for the purposes of tinnitus remediation are within the audiology scope of practice and outlined in the ASHA Preferred Practice Patterns for the Profession of Audiology.[3] When it comes to recommendations related to use of supplements or medications to improve sleep, this should be directed by the patient's primary care physician or referring provider. In this case, our patient was seen by an interdisciplinary team for concussion, so sleep assessment and intervention was already in progress.

4. *Would the inclusion of ARTs add diagnostic value to this assessment?*
   DD exhibited an asymmetry (three test frequencies of > 10 dB) in the left ear. ARTs are a valuable tool for assessment of cranial nerve path integrity to make appropriate referrals if a retrocochlear lesion is suspected. In this case, DD was referred from neurology as part of the concussion clinic and she received a CT scan during her admittance to the ER following the accident. It is important to note that

documentation of a computed tomography (CT) or magnetic resonance imaging (MRI) does not mean the imaging was done for the purpose or view needed to investigate otologic injuries. Although the presence of normal ARTs in this case would have added potential diagnostic value, absence of ARTs would not help differentiate the locus of injury. DD's audiological results were reviewed by the neurologist directing her care, and subsequent imaging ruled out additional otologic concerns beyond the tinnitus. The potential for AR activator tones to exacerbate tinnitus or provoke a sensation of sound intolerance must be considered prior to undertaking the test.

5. *If a patient is managing their tinnitus well with TRT, should they continue using it indefinitely?*
   TRT efficacy data supports the continued use of sound therapy for at least 18 months.[11] Beyond that point, patients vary greatly in the time needed to continue TRT before an acceptable level of habituation is reached.[12] Our TRT program includes a plan for patients to begin reducing wear time after 18 months with increased focus on progressive muscle relaxation (PMR) and masking acutely when needed. The TRT Trial data in 2019[20] showed about 50% of patients experienced a reduction in tinnitus using TRT, partial TRT, or standard of care (SOC) treatment.[23] SOC treatment involves basic counseling of tinnitus and is not at the depth or breadth outlined in TRT. If a patient is not experiencing improvement with 18 months of TRT, we change our treatment program knowing that half of our patients may not benefit from it and another treatment option may be more beneficial in a given case.

6.5 Recommendations and Outcomes

DD was prescribed Desyrel by the team physician for anxiety-related sleep disturbance. Although she reported tinnitus during waking hours only and it had no interference with sleep, she was instructed on PMR techniques to aid in relaxation for sleep. She was referred for cognitive behavioral therapy (CBT) with psychology and started TRT + mild amplification for the left ear in our clinic. She initiated an app-based masker when driving; the radio was reported as bothersome, and she acquired filtered earplugs (ETY plugs) for sporting events. She began sound enrichment at home using the masker-app and classical music at a comfortable volume. One-month follow-up visit THI score was 62 and TFI score 78. Three-month follow-up THI score was 48 and TFI 50. She attended a first visit with CBT and decided not to pursue it. DD reported to us that she received good strategies for working through her anxiety and was able to practice techniques at home. Her 6-month concussion symptom checklist score was 33, THI 36, and TFI 48. At this point, she was taking Melatonin for sleep; no longer Desyrel and reportedly managing tinnitus with the TRT device/streamed masking sounds during the day with good success. She was emotional at this visit, expressing gratitude and reporting her symptoms had improved dramatically. At this point we recommended she continue TRT for at least 18 months before starting her sound therapy reduction plan.

6.6 Key Points

- Head injuries complicate the treatment of tinnitus and these patients often require team-based care. Without the work of neurology and psychology, this patient might not have been successful in managing her tinnitus under the extreme anxiety and lack of sleep she experienced.
- Information counseling is an important component of TRT, even in simplified applications of the TRT process. There is evidence that using the TRT process with shorter counseling sessions can lead to successful outcomes.[1] In this case, the etiology of tinnitus and comorbid conditions warranted more extensive counseling at each visit. It is important to consider every patient and be well prepared in a tinnitus clinic to have flexibility.

References

[1] Aazh H, Moore BC, Glasberg BR. Simplified form of tinnitus retraining therapy in adults: a retrospective study. BMC Ear Nose Throat Disord. 2008; 8:7

[2] Alster J, Shemesh Z, Ornan M, Attias J. Sleep disturbance associated with chronic tinnitus. Biol Psychiatry. 1993; 34(1–2):84–90

[3] ASHA Working Group. Preferred practice patterns for the profession of audiology. 2006, December. https://www.asha.org/policy/PP2006–00274/

[4] Beck AT, Guth D, Steer RA, Ball R. Screening for major depression disorders in medical inpatients with the Beck Depression Inventory for Primary Care. Behav Res Ther. 1997; 35(8):785–791

[5] Bergemalm PO. Progressive hearing loss after closed head injury: a predictable outcome. Acta Otolaryngol. 2003; 123 (7):836–845

[6] Bergemalm PO, Borg E. Peripheral and central audiological sequelae of closed head injury: function, activity, participation and quality of life. Audiol Med. 2005; 3(3):185–198

[7] Choi MS, Shin SO, Yeon JY, Choi YS, Kim J, Park SK. Clinical characteristics of labyrinthine concussion. Korean J Audiol. 2013; 17(1):13–17

[8] Chorney SR, Suryadevara AC, Nicholas BD. Audiovestibular symptoms as predictors of prolonged sports-related concussion among NCAA athletes. Laryngoscope. 2017; 127(12):2850–2853

[9] Folmer RL, Griest SE. Chronic tinnitus resulting from head or neck injuries. Laryngoscope. 2003; 113(5):821–827

[10] Frommer LJ, Gurka KK, Cross KM, Ingersoll CD, Comstock RD, Saliba SA. Sex differences in concussion symptoms of high school athletes. J Athl Train. 2011; 46(1):76–84

[11] Jastreboff PJ, Jastreboff MM. Tinnitus Retraining Therapy (TRT) as a method for treatment of tinnitus and hyperacusis patients. J Am Acad Audiol. 2000; 11(3):162–177

[12] Jastreboff PJ. 25 years of tinnitus retraining therapy. HNO. 2015; 63(4):307–311

[13] Kreuzer PM, Landgrebe M, Schecklmann M, Staudinger S, Langguth B, TRI Database Study Group. Trauma-associated tinnitus: audiological, demographic and clinical characteristics. PLoS One. 2012; 7(9):e45599

[14] Lin CE, Chen LF, Chou PH, Chung CH. Increased prevalence and risk of anxiety disorders in adults with tinnitus: A population-based study in Taiwan. Gen Hosp Psychiatry. 2018; 50:131–136

[15] Lovell MR, Collins MW. Neuropsychological assessment of the college football player. J Head Trauma Rehabil. 1998; 13 (2):9–26

[16] Meikle MB, Henry JA, Griest SE, et al. The tinnitus functional index: development of a new clinical measure for chronic, intrusive tinnitus. Ear Hear. 2012; 33(2):153–176

[17] Newman CW, Jacobson GP, Spitzer JB. Development of the Tinnitus Handicap Inventory. Arch Otolaryngol Head Neck Surg. 1996; 122(2):143–148

[18] Nölle C, Todt I, Seidl RO, Ernst A. Pathophysiological changes of the central auditory pathway after blunt trauma of the head. J Neurotrauma. 2004; 21(3):251–258

[19] Ohhashi G, Tani S, Murakami S, Kamio M, Abe T, Ohtuki J. Problems in health management of professional boxers in Japan. Br J Sports Med. 2002; 36(5):346–352, discussion 353

[20] The Tinnitus Retraining Therapy Trial Research Group. Effect of tinnitus retraining therapy vs standard of care on tinnitus-related quality of life: a randomized clinical trial. JAMA Otolaryngol Head Neck Surg. Published online May 23, 2019. DOI: 10.1001/jamaoto.2019.0821

[21] Vibert D, Häusler R. Acute peripheral vestibular deficits after whiplash injuries. Ann Otol Rhinol Laryngol. 2003; 112(3):246–251

[22] Whiteneck GG, Cuthbert JP, Corrigan JD, Bogner JA. Risk of negative outcomes after traumatic brain injury: a statewide population-based survey. J Head Trauma Rehabil. 2016; 31 (1):E43–E54

[23] Tinnitus Retraining Therapy Trial Research Group, Scherer RW, Formby C. Effect of tinnitus retraining therapy vs standard of care on tinnitus-related quality of life: a randomized clinical trial. JAMA Otolaryngol Head Neck Surg. 2019 Jul 1;145(7):597–608. doi: 10.1001/jamaoto.2019.0821

7 Tinnitus in a Case of Meniere's Disease

Lauren Mann

7.1 Clinical History and Presentation

GM is a 56-year-old female who first presented to our clinic with reports of right ear tonal tinnitus, vertigo with emesis, and sudden hearing loss she attributed to significant weight loss following lap band surgery. Results from the first evaluation in our office indicated mild-to-moderate sensorineural hearing loss (SNHL) with asymmetrically worse hearing in the right ear (▸ Fig. 7.1).

Her speech testing results were all consistent with her audiogram and reported history where she reported no difficulty understanding speech in quiet or noisy conditions (▸ Fig. 7.2).

At that time, tinnitus was pitch-matched to 6.5 kHz with reference tones played in the left, better hearing ear and confirmed in the right tinnitus ear (▸ Fig. 7.3). The tinnitus presentation was consistent with her history of significant factory and motorcycle noise exposure. Acoustic reflex thresholds (ARTs) were absent, bilaterally, but tympanometry was normal (▸ Fig. 7.4). Her Tinnitus Handicap Inventory (THI)[1] at this visit was 32, which is considered mild.

We referred GM to an ear, nose, and throat (ENT) physician for unilateral tinnitus, vertigo, absent acoustic reflex thresholds (ARTs), and asymmetrical hearing loss. One year later, she returned to our clinic after being diagnosed with Meniere's disease (MD, idiopathic endolymphatic hydrops) as supported with large SP/AP ratio during an eCochG.[2] GM was referred back to our clinic at this point for severe tinnitus after the right ear progressed to a flat, moderately severe SNHL and she had reached burnout of her vestibular symptoms.

The tinnitus case history and interview included a THI[1] score of 76 (severe), a Tinnitus Functional Index (TFI)[3] score of 88 (severe), and Beck Depression Inventory Screening PC[4] score of 10 (normal to mild). She reported significant distress with the ongoing tinnitus, difficulty hearing, and reported thoughts of suicide; she gave an example plan. She noted that she felt helpless with her tinnitus and became significantly depressed when her vertigo resolved but tinnitus did not. At this point in the interview, GM was immediately escorted to the emergency room with her permission and was admitted to the hospital for psychiatric monitoring. Subsequent outpatient psychiatry reports indicated

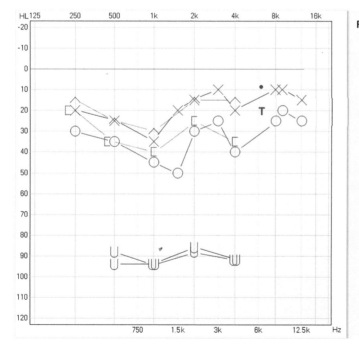

Fig. 7.1 Initial audiogram.

R	SRT	30		AC	Spondee Word List
L	SRT	15		AC	Spondee Word List
R	UCL	90		AC	Rainbow Passage
L	UCL	95		AC	Rainbow Passage
R	WRS	70 [50]	100.0%	AC	NU-6 List 1A
L	WRS	55 [35]	92.0%	AC	NU-6 List 2A

Fig. 7.2 Initial speech testing.

Tinnitus Evaluation	Stimulus Ear		
Visit One	Right	Binaural	Left
Pitch Matching	T 6500 Hz		T 6500 Hz
Loudness Matching			T 12 SL
Hearing Threshold	• 30 HL		• 8 HL
Masking Noise Threshold	12 HL	4 HL	2 HL
Minimum Masking Level (MML)	24 SL (36 HL)	32 SL (36 HL)	
Maskability	Complete	Complete	
Residual Inhibition	8 s		
Inhibition Characteristic	Complete		

Note: Reduced gain post RI

Fig. 7.3 Initial tinnitus evaluation.

instructions on progressive muscle relaxation (PMR), medication for clinical depression, and permission to proceed with audiological evaluation and management of tinnitus.

At her next evaluation, 1 month later, her new THI score was 72 (severe), TFI score was 80 (severe), and Beck Depression Inventory Screening PC score was 3 (normal). She reported feeling more equipped to handle the constant tinnitus but was still very disturbed by it and was looking forward to a "cure."

7.2 Audiological Evaluation

GM's pure-tone audiogram showed a flat, moderately severe SNHL in the right ear and a moderate loss rising to normal hearing in the high frequencies for the left ear. Uncomfortable loudness levels (UCLs) were assessed using warble tones from 500 to 4 kHz in each ear and results between 100 and 110 dB HL indicated an expected dynamic range in each ear (▶ Fig. 7.5).

Speech recognition thresholds (SRTs) were established at 65 dB HL in the right and 25 dB HL in the left ear. Word recognition was 52% at 95 dB HL (75 dBEML) in the right and 90% at 55 dB HL in the left when presented with NU-6 Ordered-by-Difficulty lists one and two (▶ Fig. 7.6).

Tympanometry was normal for both ears, and ARTs were repeated to rule out test error since we expected ARTs in the better hearing ear. They were again absent bilaterally in all conditions (▶ Fig. 7.7).

Tinnitus was matched to a 9-kHz tone at 14 dB SL re: pure-tone threshold at 9 kHz, with reference stimuli in the left ear. Her tinnitus pitch was higher than her previous match of 6.5 kHz one year prior. Her minimal masking level (MML) was found in the right ear with 14 dB SL re: white noise threshold. She experienced 12 seconds of residual inhibition following a one-minute presentation of white noise at 10 dB SL re: MML and reported substantial reduction in tinnitus volume for the duration of the visit (▶ Fig. 7.8).

7.3 Questions for the Reader

1. Is GM's tinnitus typical for Meniere's disease?
2. Given the fluctuations of hearing and tinnitus seen in Meniere's disease, what considerations

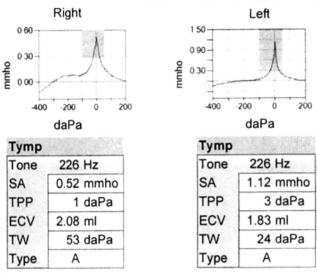

Fig. 7.4 Initial immitance.

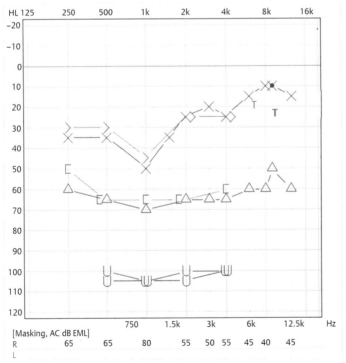

Fig. 7.5 Current speech testing.

Speech	SDT		SRT		WRS / SRS 1				WRS / SRS 2				MCL	UCL
	dB HL	[m]	dB HL	[m]	%	dB HL	[m]	S/N	%	dB HL	[m]	S/N	dB HL	dB HL
Right			65		52	95	[75]								100
Left			25		90	55									
Bin															
Note	¹File NU-6 List 1A						²File NU-6 List 2A								
Aided															
Note	1						2								

Fig. 7.6 Current audiogram.

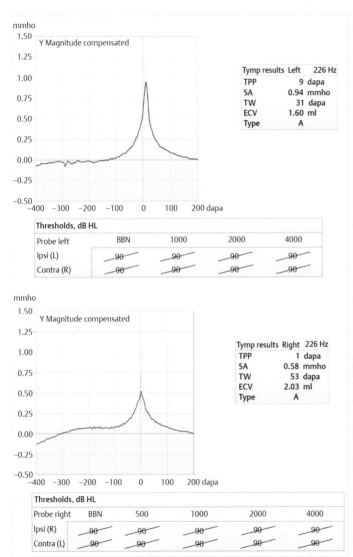

Fig. 7.7 Current immitance.

Tymp results Left   226 Hz
TPP   9 dapa
SA   0.94 mmho
TW   31 dapa
ECV   1.60 ml
Type   A

Thresholds, dB HL

Probe left	BBN	1000	2000	4000
Ipsi (L)	90	90	90	90
Contra (R)	90	90	90	90

Tymp results Right 226 Hz
TPP   1 dapa
SA   0.58 mmho
TW   53 dapa
ECV   2.03 ml
Type   A

Thresholds, dB HL

Probe right	BBN	500	1000	2000	4000
Ipsi (R)	90	90	90	90	90
Contra (L)	90	90	90	90	90

Tinnitus Evaluation	Stimulus Ear		
Visit Two	Right	Binaural	Left
Pitch Matching	T 9000 Hz		T 9000 Hz
Loudness Matching			T 14 SL
Hearing Threshold			• 10 HL
Masking Noise Threshold	34 HL	-6 HL	-4 HL
Minimum Masking Level (MML)	14 SL (48 HL)	36 SL (30 HL)	
Maskability	Complete	Complete	
Residual Inhibition	12 s	3 s	
Inhibition Characteristic	Complete	Complete	

Note: Post RI gain reduced binaural and right side

Fig. 7.8 Current tinnitus evaluation.

are needed for amplification and/or sound therapy?

3. What are the roles and responsibilities of the audiologist when a patient's safety is uncertain?

7.4 Discussion of Questions for the Reader

1. *Is GM's tinnitus typical for Meniere's disease?*
   Tinnitus from MD has been characterized as a "low-pitched buzz or roar" since the 1960s.[5] GM's tinnitus is more consistent with the high-frequency tonal tinnitus associated with SNHL. GM's history of significant noise exposure could be contributing to this atypical presentation.

2. *Given the fluctuations of hearing and tinnitus seen in Meniere's disease, what considerations are needed for amplification and/or sound therapy?*
   The tinnitus etiology of MD does not exclude patients from Tinnitus Retraining Therapy (TRT) candidacy, but it is important that the underlying MD be medically managed under the care of a physician prior to initiating any type of audiological intervention for tinnitus.[6]
   The configuration, asymmetry, and fluctuation seen in MD present a significant challenge for appropriate fitting of amplification and/or TRT. Patients may benefit from the use of multiple programs, flexibility of gain, and directionality as accessed wirelessly, and consideration of midspeech frequency gain.[7]

3. *What are the roles and responsibilities of the audiologist when a patient's safety is uncertain?*
   Aazh and Moore[8] found 13% of tinnitus patients

reporting suicidal ideations. There is no federal-mandated reporting of suicidal thoughts as there is for suspected child and elder abuse, but many states follow similar guidance for mandated reporting. As the provider, be aware of facility protocol, and the state laws for mandated reporting. Determination of suicidal risk is not in the scope of practice for audiology; however, some intake forms (e.g., the Tinnitus Reactions Questionnaire)[9] question the patient regarding suicide ideation. Screening for mental illness and suicidal thoughts may assist mental health professionals and lead to earlier intervention. Develop a protocol that includes appropriate reporting hotline numbers, facility mental health protocols, and when to send patients to emergency services.[10]

7.5 Recommendations and Outcomes

GM was counseled on the importance of hearing protection at work and was fit with custom ear-plugs. The earplugs were designed as silicone canal-style molds for use at work and while wearing her motorcycle helmet. Although a full shell style earplug is appropriate for industrial noise, the canal style allowed her to comfortably remove her helmet without pain or pressure from the ear-plugs. She was encouraged to begin a sound en-richment program per our clinical protocol and was re-instructed on PMR practices. GM was fit with a unilateral receiver-in-canal (RIC) device with sound therapy and extended bandwidth in the right ear. She was given amplification with a high-pass filtered sound therapy set at mixing ratio in the automatic setting for daily use. She was given two masker options (pink noise and ocean waves) in manual positions for immediate acute relief. The device included wireless connectivity to her iPhone allowing GM the ability to adjust volume of amplification and sound therapy stimuli on her own. This particular model included remote-programming capability in the event that a more dramatic change was needed in amplification or sound therapy before GM could be seen in the clinic. Her 1-month follow-up visit THI score was 22 (mild) and TFI was 18 (mild); she reported substantial benefit with the device. She continued psychiatric services and medication for clinical depression per her medical report from primary care. GM did not return for the 3-month follow-up reporting little to no tinnitus perception with the device in place and successful management with PMR/masking at night. She reported her tinnitus was mostly controlled with sound therapy and amplification except for "flare ups" with extreme stress or lack of sleep. We encouraged GM to continue using sound therapy for 18 months and scheduled follow-up phone calls at 6 months and 1 year. She returned for testing at 1 year and her hearing was stable. Tinnitus was not present at the time of the appointment and was not evaluated. At this point, the automatic sound therapy was moved to a manual program position along with her maskers, and she continued with amplification only. She continues regular counseling and has returned for a second annual follow-up with no evidence of tinnitus disturbance per our tinnitus inventories, although she reports continued mild flare-ups with stress or noise exposure.

7.6 Key Points

- MD presents unique challenges to the management of tinnitus due to fluctuation and pitch of typical tinnitus symptoms. MD does not preclude additional etiology of tinnitus, so it is important to consider the patient's entire medical and environmental history when developing a tinnitus management plan.
- Although only a small proportion of clinical patients may express thoughts of suicide, it is important to know your role as the provider and have a plan prepared. The use of appropriate questionnaires and case history questioning is vital to learning of any suicidal ideations.

References

[1] Newman CW, Jacobson GP, Spitzer JB. Development of the Tinnitus Handicap Inventory. Arch Otolaryngol Head Neck Surg. 1996; 122(2):143–148

[2] Ferraro JA, Durrant JD. Electrocochleography in the evaluation of patients with Ménière's disease/endolymphatic hydrops. J Am Acad Audiol. 2006; 17(1):45–68

[3] Meikle MB, Henry JA, Griest SE, et al. The Tinnitus Functional Index: development of a new clinical measure for chronic, intrusive tinnitus. Ear Hear. 2012; 33(2):153–176

[4] Beck AT, Guth D, Steer RA, Ball R. Screening for major depression disorders in medical inpatients with the Beck Depression Inventory for Primary Care. Behav Res Ther. 1997; 35(8):785–791

[5] Nodar RH, Graham JT. An investigation of frequency characteristics of tinnitus associated with Meniere's disease. Arch Otolaryngol. 1965; 82:28–31

[6] Jastreboff PJ, Jastreboff MM. Tinnitus Retraining Therapy (TRT) as a method for treatment of tinnitus and hyperacusis patients. J Am Acad Audiol. 2000; 11(3):162–177

[7] Valente M, Mispagel K, Valente LM, Hullar T. Problems and solutions for fitting amplification to patients with Ménière's disease. J Am Acad Audiol. 2006; 17(1):6–15

[8] Aazh H, Moore BCJ. Thoughts about suicide and self-harm in patients with tinnitus and hyperacusis. J Am Acad Audiol. 2018; 29(3):255–261

[9] Wilson PH, Henry J, Bowen M, Haralambous G. Tinnitus reaction questionnaire: psychometric properties of a measure of distress associated with tinnitus. J Speech Hear Res. 1991; 34(1):197–201

[10] Donaher J, Scott LA. Be prepared to help at-risk clients. ASHA Lead. 2014; 19(5):52–58

8 A Case of a Normal Hearing with Tinnitus

Wan Syafira Ishak

This is a case report of a 38-year-old female who presented with normal hearing bilaterally and high-pitched tinnitus in the left ear.

8.1 Clinical History and Description

AZ was a 38-year-old female when first referred to the audiology clinic with a complaint of reduced hearing in the left ear that developed suddenly during the first trimester of her pregnancy. She expressed no difficulty in one-to-one communication but reported problems following conversations in noisy and other adverse listening condition. The hearing difficulty was accompanied by a high-pitched tinnitus in the left ear, and she reported reduced tolerance for loud sounds. AZ reported no history of dizziness or vertigo and denied otalgia, otorrhea, and aural fullness. She had a history of Bell's palsy on the left side a few months before her pregnancy from which she fully recovered.

8.2 Audiological Testing

On otoscopy examination, both ear canals were clear and tympanic membranes were intact. Pure-tone audiometry (▶ Fig. 8.1) showed normal thresholds in both ears, with the left ear thresholds being slightly worse than the right. Speech recognition thresholds (SRTs) in quiet were at 15 dB HL (hearing level) in the right ear and 20 dB HL in the left ear indicating good test reliability.

Immittance audiometry revealed type A tympanograms bilaterally, indicative of normal middle ear function. Ipsilateral and contralateral acoustic reflex thresholds (ARTs) were not conducted due to patient reports of loudness intolerance. A transient-evoked otoacoustic emissions (TEOAE) test showed robust emissions in both ears. Tinnitus was pitch-matched at a frequency of 1.5 kHz.

8.3 Questions for the Reader

1. Based on the initial audiological results, what would be the most likely pathology?
2. What findings would raise suspicion of retrocochlear lesion?
3. What further audiological testing should be recommended?
4. Is the use of acoustic reflex testing warranted in this case?

8.4 Discussion of Questions for the Reader

1. *Based on the initial audiological results, what would be the most likely pathology?*
   This patient presented with a normal pure-tone audiometry, normal SRTs, type A tympanograms, and robust TEOAEs, bilaterally. Thus, given the normal findings, the cause for tinnitus and difficulty hearing in noise cannot be explained with the initial audiological results. The patient could have a subclinical

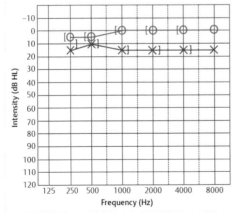

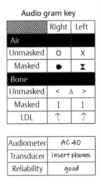

Fig. 8.1 Initial audiogram and tympanometry results of AZ.

processing abnormality that requires further assessment for differential diagnosis. Although tinnitus has long been associated with hearing loss, there are patients with normal audiometric findings who experience bothersome tinnitus. According to literature, approximately 8–10% of tinnitus population present with normal hearing thresholds.

2. *What findings would raise suspicion of retrocochlear lesion?*

Having a unilateral tinnitus may be the red flag for retrocochlear lesion. A study by Choi et al[1] found that unilateral tinnitus occurred in about 80% of confirmed acoustic neuroma cases. Based on the patient's audiological results, the only remarkable finding was slightly elevated thresholds at three adjacent frequencies (2,000, 4,000, and 8,000 Hz) in the left ear as compared to the right ear. Typically, a slight asymmetry of 15 dB at high frequencies may not cause any concern due to the typical effects of noise exposure. However, history of noise exposure or noise trauma was not indicated by the patient. Thus, the presence of a slight asymmetric hearing at high frequencies raised the suspicion of retrocochlear lesion. Nonetheless, having an asymmetric hearing and unilateral tinnitus alone would be insufficient evidence for the patient to receive a more sensitive diagnostic assessment such as a magnetic resonance imaging (MRI) scan. Further audiological assessments are warranted to further support the suspicion of retrocochlear lesion. In addition, the patient did not present with the classical symptoms of retrocochlear lesion such as aural fullness and balance problem; thus, further assessment facilitating differential diagnosis is crucial.

3. *What further audiological testing should be recommended?*

Several options are possible. Behavioral assessment using the thresholds equalizing noise (TEN) test could be conducted in order to assess cochlear integrity. Auditory brainstem response (ABR) test could be performed to rule out retrocochlear lesion; however, the ABR's sensitivity is proportional to the size of the tumor. Despite the diagnostic limitations of ABRs, the need to limit health costs as well as the difficulty in gaining access to MRI (at least in our setting) have led to this test being considered as a means of screening for retrocochlear lesion.

4. *Is the use of acoustic reflex testing warranted in this case?*

Some tinnitus patients may experience hypersensitivity toward sound. Meanwhile, in some patients, exposure to loud sound can exacerbate the tinnitus. Therefore, acoustic reflex testing, although an important element of differential diagnostic assessment, should be reconsidered in some instances. In this case, acoustic reflex testing is important to help in differential diagnosis. However, in this case, acoustic reflex testing should be eliminated or delayed, as the patient has intolerance toward loud noise. Alternative tests should be performed to help in differential diagnosis.

8.5 Additional Testing

8.5.1 Audiological

The TEN test was conducted with this patient. A compatible CD player was connected to a two-channel Grason Stadler GSI 60 audiometer with TDH 39 headphones. The left output of the CD player was connected to the left / External A input of the audiometer and the right output was fed to the External B. Then the left (External A) input was selected as Channel 1 and the right (External B) input was selected as Channel 2. The test was calibrated using track 1 of the CD prior to the testing. Track 1 contains the calibrating tone that is used to set the VU meter readings of both channels of the audiometer to 0 dB. Later, the two channels were mixed and directed to the desired ear for testing. In other words, the patient will hear the test tone and the noise in the same ear. The intensity level of the test tone was controlled by Channel 2 of the audiometer. Then, the masking noise level was set at a fixed 50 dB HL/ERB$_N$ using the Channel 1 control dial. The patient was instructed to respond only if she heard testing tones, as she ignored the noise. The masked thresholds were measured for each frequency using tracks 2 to 8 of the CD while the noise was playing continuously. The final step size was adjusted in 2-dB steps. A cochlear dead region for a particular frequency was indicated by a masked threshold of 10 dB or more than the masking noise level. Abnormal results were found at 1, 1.5, 3, and 4 kHz on the left ear suggesting abnormal function of inner hair cells and/or neural function (▶ Table 8.1). ABR test with a standard stimulus rate revealed normal peak and interpeak latencies in the right ear. However, there was

Table 8.1 TEN test results for subject AZ with the TEN level set at 50 dB HL/ERB$_N$

	Frequency (kHz)						
	0.5	0.75	1.0	1.5	2.0	3.0	4.0
Right ear							
• Absolute threshold (dB HL)	5	5	0	0	0	5	0
• Masked threshold (dB HL)	50	50	50	50	50	50	50
Left ear							
• Absolute threshold (dB HL)	10	10	15	20	15	15	15
• Masked threshold (dB HL)	50	52	60*	62*	54	62*	60*

Abbreviation: TEN, thresholds equalizing noise.
* indicates abnormal results.

absence of wave V at 70 dBnHL (normalized hearing level) in the left ear.

8.5.2 Radiology

The MRI (▶ Fig. 8.2) revealed a large acoustic neuroma on the left cellebellar pontine (CP) angle. It was 2.95 × 2.4 cm in size. The tumor compressed the brainstem cisternal portion of the VIIIth cranial nerve.

8.6 Final Diagnosis and Recommended Treatment

The definitive diagnosis for AZ was unilateral left acoustic neuroma. Treatment options for an acoustic neuroma case include active monitoring, microsurgery, stereotactic radiation therapy, stereotactic radiosurgery (Gamma Knife), and proton beam therapy. The treatment options were presented to the patient. Due to the size of the tumor, the neurotologist recommended microsurgery or stereotactic radiosurgery. After considering the advantages and disadvantages of each option, AZ chose to undergo stereotactic radiosurgery.

8.7 Outcome

AZ was seen for follow-up audiological examination 6 months after the stereotactic radiosurgery. The otoscopic examination revealed clear ear canal with intact tympanic membranes bilaterally. The tympanometry showed ear canal volumes, peak pressure, and static admittance, all were within normal range bilaterally. Pure-tone audiometry results (▶ Fig. 8.3) for the right ear showed

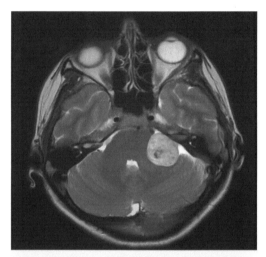

Fig. 8.2 The axial magnetic resonance imaging (MRI) section of the internal auditory meatus. There is 2.95 × 2.4 cm of acoustic neuroma at the left cerebellopontine angle compressing the brainstem and cisternal portion of the VIIIth cranial nerve.

thresholds within normal limit at all frequencies tested. These thresholds were consistent with the initial audiogram findings. However, the audiometry results for the left ear revealed a mild sensorineural hearing loss from 1,000 Hz through the higher frequencies. The thresholds were slightly decreased and the asymmetry hearing became more significant than the initial visit. This result was expected as stereotactic radiation may cause the tumor to swell prior to shrinkage. The radiation may also cause damage to the peripheral organs, which may result in worsening hearing thresholds and tinnitus. AZ, however, denied any worsening of tinnitus. AZ performed within normal

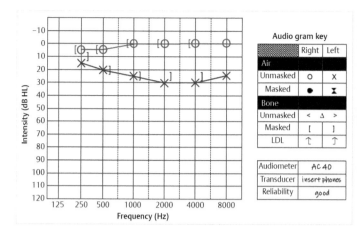

Fig. 8.3 AZ's audiological results 6 months after stereotactic radiosurgery for an acoustic neuroma in the left ear.

percentiles for both quiet and noise front conditions of Hearing in Noise Test (HINT). Although AZ had mild sensorineural hearing loss in the left ear, she still had bilateral functional hearing; thus, an amplification device was not recommended at this point. Effective communication strategies were suggested to the patient.

Reference

[1] Choi KJ, Sajisevi MB, Kahmke RR, Kaylie DM. Incidence of retrocochlear pathology found on MRI in patients with non-pulsatile tinnitus. Otol Neurotol. 2015; 36(10):1730–1734

Suggested Readings

Moore BC. Dead regions in the cochlea: conceptual foundations, diagnosis, and clinical applications. Ear Hear. 2004; 25(2):98–116

Schaette R, McAlpine D. Tinnitus with a normal audiogram: physiological evidence for hidden hearing loss and computational model. J Neurosci. 2011; 31(38):13452–13457

Schmidt RJ, Sataloff RT, Newman J, Spiegel JR, Myers DL. The sensitivity of auditory brainstem response testing for the diagnosis of acoustic neuromas. Arch Otolaryngol Head Neck Surg. 2001; 127(1):19–22

Theodosopoulos PV, Pensak ML. Contemporary management of acoustic neuromas. Laryngoscope. 2011; 121(6):1133–1137

Weisz N, Hartmann T, Dohrmann K, Schlee W, Norena A. High-frequency tinnitus without hearing loss does not mean absence of deafferentation. Hear Res. 2006; 222(1–2):108–114

9 Functional Audiogenic Seizure

David M. Baguley

9.1 Clinical History/Description

Following referral from her family doctor, a 50-year-old woman (MA) attended a specialist Tinnitus and Hyperacusis outpatient clinic in the United Kingdom. MA was accompanied by her husband, and she was utilizing a wheel chair. It was noted that she was using noise-cancelling headphones in the clinic waiting room. Her primary complaint was 4 years of frequent, at least daily, sound-induced seizures which lasted several minutes, and during which MA reported "I am not myself." The appearance of the seizure was of strong upper body and neck muscle spasm, facial grimacing, and eye closure. Trigger sounds were not particularly intense, nor perceived as overly loud, but rather were unexpected and intrusive. For example, while at the clinic, a seizure was triggered by a colleague whistling outside the non-sound-treated clinic room.

MA experienced a number of nonauditory symptoms. She had been diagnosed previously with chronic fatigue syndrome, restless leg syndrome, obstructive sleep apnea, and depression. Her family physician diagnosed many of these conditions. MA had consulted some specialists but described her consultations as having not gone well.

Medications of note were sertraline (which MA described as helpful for her mood), nortriptyline, and betahistine. MA was concerned that the use of nortriptyline was exacerbating her seizures.

The impact of the sound-induced seizures was distressing, and served to render her housebound, as even with hearing protection and/or noise cancelling headphones, environmental sounds on a social or shopping trip caused debilitating and embarrassing seizures. This sound sensitivity had caused her to be retired on health grounds from her work as a preschool teaching assistant.

9.2 Audiologic Testing

Otoscopy was normal. At the initial visit, pure-tone audiometry was not performed, as there was no medical/nursing coverage to support MA in the event of a large seizure. When testing was performed at a subsequent clinic attendance, all thresholds were found to be within normal limits.

9.3 Questions for the Reader

1. What features of this case are convergent and divergent with hyperacusis, as it is generally understood?
2. What putative diagnosis might be made and to whom might onward referral be made to confirm this?
3. Is there a role for audiologic management in a case such as this?

9.4 Discussion of Questions for the Reader

1. *What features of this case are convergent and divergent with hyperacusis, as it is generally understood?*

   Hyperacusis refers to the situation in which every day environmental sound is perceived as overwhelmingly loud or intense.[1] The term "hyperacusis" is sometimes used in conjunction with the phrase "decreased sound tolerance" or "reduced sound tolerance." This particular case is an example for which the term "hyperacusis" and these phrases are not synonymous. MA did not perceive her seizure triggers as intense; rather, it was their unexpected and abrupt nature that was characteristic. This is certainly an example of the abnormal tolerance of sound, but not of hyperacusis.

   It should also be noted, however, that the behavioral consequences of these audiogenic seizures map closely onto those in standard hyperacusis, specifically the avoidance of sound, and withdrawal from social and professional situations in which one might be exposed to sound. In addition, both symptoms can lead to anxiety and fear about sound exposure. Finally, the (over)reliance upon hearing protection is common to both.

2. *What putative diagnosis might be made and to whom might onward referral be made to confirm this?*

   There is a new paradigm regarding medically unexplained symptoms in the field of Neurology, entitled Functional Neurological Disorders (FNDs), defined as follows:

   "The presentation of neurologic symptoms that are internally inconsistent or incongruent with the patterns of pathophysiologic disease"[2] (following DSM-5).[3]

At the outset of this discussion, it is important to note that the neurological community uses the word *functional* in quite a different manner than the audiological community. For an audiologist, *functional* carries an implication of malingering or pretense, and there may be an assumption of intentionality. In a hybrid, audiologic/psychologic model of nonorganic hearing loss (NOHL), Austen and Lynch[4] considered the factors of motivation, gain (benefit), the degree of intentionality, and consistency of test responses. The possibility that NOHL might have a psychological component was also raised. For the psychologic community, *functional* applies to genuine and authentic symptoms in the absence of any identifiable pathophysiological process. FND includes such debilitating symptoms as movement disorders, tremor, coma, and visual disturbances[6], essentially the full gamut of neurologic symptoms. The application of the FND perspective to auditory disorders was undertaken by Baguley et al,[5] considering NOHL, tinnitus, and hyperacusis as having the potential for attributes of FND.

The experiences of MA were suggestive of an FND component when reviewed in the Tinnitus and Hyperacusis clinic. No hearing loss or audiological abnormality was detected, and the nature of the seizures appeared to the team to have a marked dissociative element. The possibility that her seizures were nonepileptic in nature was proposed. A referral was made to the University Hospital multidisciplinary FND clinic.

3. *Is there a role for audiologic management in a case such as this?*

Several features of this case indicate a role for audiologic management. First, referrals of this sort may be made to audiology-based hyperacusis services, which need to be aware of the FND perspective, and able to make appropriate onward referral(s). While the treatment of FND often includes psychotherapy, and in the case of movement disorders, physical therapy, in the event of audiogenic seizure the process of giving the patient an element of control over their symptoms can, in the case of sound, involve audiologic management, as will be seen below.

9.5 Final Diagnosis and Recommended Treatment

The multidisciplinary FND clinic team members concurred that these audiogenic seizures were nonepileptic, and they were confident that a substantial FND component was evident. They noted that sound is not a common trigger of nonepileptic seizure.[7] The diagnosis of FND was shared with MA, who felt that this was a very encouraging development. The other nonaudiologic symptoms/conditions, although outside the scope of this report, were also discussed with MA. The use of nortriptyline and betahistine was discontinued.

MA returned to the audiology clinic with her diagnosis, and a program of gradual reduction of hearing protection and an increase in sound exposure was embarked upon. This was self-directed and informal but discussed in detail with the audiology team.

An immediate reduction in the occurrence of seizures was evident. From the daily seizures initially indicated, MA reported two seizures in a 3-month period, both of which had been triggered by significant noise. She reported this improvement as a result of ceasing nortriptyline, although the FND team could not affirm her observation, as, in their view, the drug was more likely a trigger or exacerbating factor of seizures rather than their cause.

9.6 Outcome

On subsequent review, MA was seizure free for the prior 6 months. Use of hearing protection was now exceptional rather than routine. MA and her partner were delighted.

References

[1] Fackrell K, Potgieter I, Shekhawat GS, et al. Clinical Interventions for hyperacusis in adults: a scoping review to assess the current position and determine priorities for research. Biomed Res Int. 2017;2017:2723715. doi: 10.1155/2017/2723715

[2] Carson A, Lehn A. Epidemiology. In: Hallet M, Stone J, Carson A, eds. Functional neurologic disorders. Handbook of clinical neurology, Vol. 139, 2016:47–60

[3] American Psychiatric Association. (2013). Diagnostic and statistical manual of mental disorders (5th ed.)

[4] Austen S, Lynch C. Non-organic hearing loss redefined: understanding, categorizing and managing non-organic behaviour. Int J Audiol. 2004; 43(8):449–457

[5] Baguley DM, Cope TE, McFerran DJ. Functional auditory disorders. In: Hallet M, Stone J, Carson A, eds. Functional neurologic disorders. Handbook of clinical neurology, Vol. 139, 2016:367–378

[6] Hallett, M, Stone, J, Carson, AJ. Functional Neurological Disorders. Vol. 139. London: Academic Press; 2016

[7] Reuber M, Rawlings GH. Nonepileptic seizures—subjective phenomena. In: Hallet M, Stone J, Carson A, eds. Functional neurologic disorders. Handbook of clinical neurology, Vol. 139, 2016:283–296

Suggested Reading

O'Sullivan S. 2016. It's all in your head: stories from the frontline of psychosomatic medicine. London: Vintage

10 Postconcussive Tinnitus and Hyperacusis

Aniruddha K. Deshpande and Diana Callesano

10.1 Clinical History and Description

KG is a 39-year-old female who was involved in a motor vehicle accident in which her car was hit from behind while at a stop sign. The force of the collision caused her to lose consciousness for a few seconds. She was taken to the emergency room by ambulance where she underwent a computed tomography (CT) scan of her brain. Internal hemorrhaging was ruled out, and she was diagnosed with a moderate concussion. Immediately following the accident, KG developed bilateral multitoned tinnitus, difficulty hearing in noise, sensitivity to moderate and loud sounds, and dull headaches. Notable postconcussive changes included hearing abrupt loud sounds while falling asleep followed by periods of intense fear and insomnia, trouble concentrating, and sensitivity to light.

10.2 Audiologic Testing

10.2.1 Case History

KG works as an elementary school teacher in New York City. She returned to work part-time (3 d/wk) following the accident. KG had 30 students in her class along with two teacher's aides. She reported her classroom to be quite loud during the day especially when students congregated for group activities. Her primary complaint in the classroom was hearing her students as she could not separate their voices from the background noise. She also expressed sensitivity to the routine noise level in her classroom. KG excused herself to the teachers' lounge for brief periods to regroup when the noise became intolerable. In addition, her tinnitus was significantly heightened by the end of the workday; she reported that when she arrived home she would retreat to her bedroom and lay down for the evening. KG stated that it took about 1 day before her tinnitus returned to its baseline and her sensitivity reduced. This was problematic for her because she has three children of her own. She felt she could not meaningfully interact with them when her tinnitus was exacerbated.

10.2.2 Audiologic Evaluation

Pure-tone audiometry revealed hearing within normal limits from 250 to 4,000 Hz with a mild-to-moderate presumably sensorineural hearing loss (SNHL) from 6 to 12.5 kHz bilaterally (▶ Fig. 10.1). Speech recognition thresholds (SRTs) were obtained within normal limits and were in good agreement with the 3-frequency pure-tone average (PTA). Word recognition scores (WRS) were obtained at 40 dB SL (ref: SRT) using the Northwestern University's NU-6 Word List[1] 1A with monitored live voice. KG scored 100% in both ears consistent with an excellent score. Tympanometry revealed normal ear canal volume, static admittance, and middle ear pressure in each ear (Type A). Acoustic reflex thresholds (ARTs) could not be tested due to patient's report of sound sensitivity.

10.2.3 Tinnitus Pitch Match

Tinnitus pitch match may help the clinician define the approximate pitch of patients' tinnitus. In our clinic, various tonal stimuli are presented and the patient is asked to respond only when the external sound is similar to their subjective tinnitus. The results of this measurement may support counseling the patient and determining which sound therapy options would be most suitable for the patient. KG initially had trouble pitch-matching her tinnitus due to its multitonal nature. She was asked to focus on the two most prominent sounds for this task. KG described the primary sound as crickets in the summertime. She matched her primary tone to a continuous 6 kHz frequency-specific hearing assessment (FRESH) noise[2] and the second sound to a 1-kHz PT. The PT was heard slightly louder in the right ear while the FRESH noise was heard centrally. She also reported a steady white noise in the background that was less noticeable.

10.2.4 Tinnitus Loudness Match

Tinnitus loudness match allows the clinician to ascertain the approximate loudness of a patient's tinnitus. The test may be performed using the stimulus identified in the pitch-matching task, or a nontinnitus frequency (i.e., 500 Hz) could be matched to the tinnitus loudness. Results from the

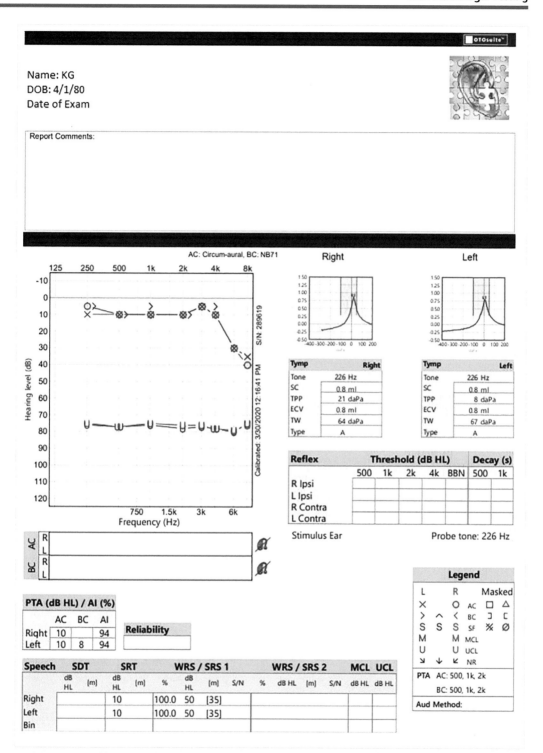

Fig. 10.1 KG's pure-tone audiometry results.

Table 10.1 KG's LDL (in dB HL) at the initial consultation using a 1-dB step size for PT across frequencies

	Frequency (Hz)							
	250	500	1000	2000	3000	4000	6000	8000
Right	75	77	75	76	76	78	79	76
Left	76	77	76	78	77	78	80	75

Abbreviations: LDL, loudness discomfort level; PT, pure tone.

two test paradigms typically reveal a far higher SL when the match to the tinnitus is made at a nontinnitus frequency. This task can be performed using a 1 or 2 dB step-size involving ascending runs to establish the estimated tinnitus loudness. The starting point is typically the patient's threshold either at the tinnitus frequency or at a nontinnitus frequency. Findings from the loudness match task may be used to guide sound therapy options to mitigate the perception of tinnitus. KG matched the dominant FRESH-noise tinnitus at 37 and 35 dB HL (or 7 and 5 dB SL ref: 6 kHz) in the left and right ears, respectively. FRESH noise is preferred for pediatric threshold estimation over the narrow band noise (NBN) due to its frequency specificity and calibration in hearing level (dB HL).[3] A similar rationale was employed to match KG's tinnitus loudness. The secondary tonal sound was perceived at 20 dB HL in both ears or 10 dB SL re: threshold at 1,000 Hz.

10.2.5 Minimum Masking Level

The minimum masking level (MML) is used to determine the amount of broadband white noise needed to completely mask the tinnitus. It is generally regarded as a more reasonable measurement than the tinnitus loudness match when establishing the level of sound to be employed in tinnitus management therapies. This measure can also be used to judge the effectiveness of sound therapy intervention as it has been shown to be a reliable estimate of tinnitus magnitude.[4] Broadband noise is presented binaurally in an ascending manner beginning at the patient's threshold. The patient is asked to signal a "stop" hand gesture when they no longer perceive their tinnitus and only the white noise is apparent. KG achieved an MML at 21 dB SL (ref: her broadband threshold of −5 dB HL).

10.2.6 Loudness Discomfort Levels

A loudness discomfort level (LDL) measurement can be used to determine if a patient presents with sound tolerance issues. This measure may be repeated throughout the course of sound therapy

intervention to reassess tolerance levels to determine whether the goal of improving the dynamic range (DR) and minimizing sound sensitivity is realized. In our clinic, this test is administered using 1 to 2 dB ascending increments and the patient is asked to raise their hand when the level has become uncomfortably loud. The patient is always reassured that this test cannot damage their hearing despite the brief presentation of high intensity sound. KG's LDLs were measured for pure tones (PT) from 250 to 8,000 Hz in each ear, showing LDLs from 75 to 80 dB HL across all frequencies (▶ Table 10.1). These results are reduced compared to typical LDL values of ≥ 100 dB HL,[5] indicating a reduced DR.

10.2.7 Residual Inhibition

Residual inhibition (RI) is a tinnitus measurement in which white noise is presented at 10 dB SL (ref: MML) in both ears for 1 to 2 minutes. This test evaluates whether a patient experiences brief suppression of their tinnitus following presentation of the noise. Prior to the RI task, KG rated her tinnitus loudness to be an 8 out of 10 (1 = very soft, 10 = very loud). After cessation of the white noise, she rated her tinnitus at a 5 out of 10. This indicates that she experienced partial tinnitus suppression post noise presentation.

10.3 Questions for the Reader

1. KG's collective symptoms point to which disorder?
2. What other auditory conditions could be playing a role in KG's case?
3. What additional tests could be used to further define KG's auditory profile?

10.4 Discussion of Questions for the Reader

1. *KG's collective symptoms point to which disorder?*
   KG's collective symptoms indicate that she may be suffering from exploding head syndrome

(EHS).[6,7] EHS is defined as a sensory parasomnia[8] wherein patients hear sudden loud sounds—described as violent bangs, thunder, or explosion—especially when falling asleep. This is typically followed by a state of confusion and fear. Patients may also experience heightened sensitivity to light, dull headaches, and tinnitus.

2. *What other auditory conditions could be playing a role in KG's case?*

KG reported difficulty hearing in noise after the motor vehicle accident. In the classroom, she consistently had trouble separating her students' voices from the ambient background noise. This collection of symptoms could point to underlying central auditory processing difficulties. Disruption to auditory processing function is a known sequela of concussions in both children and adults.[9] Although it may not be the most obvious or immediate auditory symptom, changes may occur within the auditory pathway resulting in strained communication.

3. *What additional tests could be used to further define KG's auditory profile?*

Given KG's audiometric findings, a central auditory processing test battery should be administered to identify any underlying weaknesses. Based on her symptoms, this test should include dichotic listening, temporal processing, monaural low-redundancy, and speech-in-noise measurements. Standardized tinnitus questionnaires such as the Tinnitus Functional Index (TFI)[10] and the Tinnitus Handicap Inventory (THI)[12] can also be administered to quantify the effect of tinnitus on KG's activities of daily living.

10.5 Final Diagnosis and Recommended Treatment

KG suffers from tinnitus and hyperacusis as a direct result of the motor vehicle accident. During her initial appointment, postconcussive auditory symptoms (i.e., tinnitus and hyperacusis) were discussed in detail to promote a better understanding of her current experience. It was further explained that although there is no cure for tinnitus, there are ways to manage the effects of this condition while also improving quality of life.

10.5.1 Management of Tinnitus

- Informational counseling was provided to KG including a review of the peripheral and central auditory system, the role of outer hair cell function in tinnitus perception, and involvement of the autonomic nervous system in tinnitus enhancement and hyperacusis. The tenets of Tinnitus Retraining Therapy (TRT), which has been in existence for more than 25 years, were discussed to reinforce understanding of the neurophysiologic model of tinnitus and hyperacusis.[11]

- After obtaining medical clearance, KG was fit with binaural Widex Evoke 440 Fusion 2 receiver-in-the-canal (RIC) hearing aids that were coupled to open domes. Low-gain amplification at 5 dB was provided across all frequencies. Acclimatization was set to level 3. The high-frequency gain feature was activated as the patient reported an improved sound quality with this setting turned on.

- In total, six programs were set for KG. The first program—called "Universal"—provided amplification. Five Zen programs were established. Three of the programs used Zen Aqua fractal tones. Of those three programs, the first was set to include the fractal tones plus amplification; the second to fractal tones, amplification, and white noise; and the third program was set to include only fractal tones without amplification. The two remaining Zen programs were set to White Noise: one with amplification and one without.

10.5.2 Management of Reaction to Tinnitus

- KG was counseled extensively on the process of habituation to tinnitus. The overall goal for habituation is to minimize the reaction to tinnitus with the hope that the strength of the functional connection between the auditory system and emotional centers in the CNS may be modified. If the reaction to tinnitus can be neutralized, then the probability that the tinnitus signal fades into the background increases.[12]

10.5.3 Management of Hyperacusis

- Management of hyperacusis is primarily focused on desensitization. KG implemented the white noise program in her hearing devices for settings that she perceived to be loud and overstimulating. This was specifically used during her time in the classroom. She was

Table 10.2 KG's LDL (in dB HL) at the 5-month follow-up visit measured in 1-dB step size for PT across frequencies

	Frequency (Hz)							
	250	500	1000	2000	3000	4000	6000	8000
Right	78	80	79	80	80	82	83	80
Left	79	81	81	82	80	82	83	80

Abbreviations: LDL, loudness discomfort level; PT, pure tone.

discouraged from using earplugs, except in loud environments (i.e., concerts, weddings), as this approach does not facilitate desensitization.

10.6 Outcome

KG was followed five times over the next 5 months. Initially, KG's score on the THI was 48, consistent with a moderate degree of self-perceived tinnitus impact. KG's score on the Hyperacusis Questionnaire[14] yielded a score of 72, consistent with a severe degree of impact from sound sensitivity. At her 3-month follow-up appointment, KG's score reduced to 16 on the THI and to a 36 on the Hyperacusis Questionnaire indicating an improvement in her tinnitus distress and an overall decrease in her sound sensitivity. Her pure-tone thresholds remained the same on a repeat audiogram; however, her LDLs improved slightly by 3 to 5 dB across all frequencies (▶ Table 10.2). She still expressed needing time to decompress during the school day but felt these breaks were not as necessary as they were initially. KG still reported difficulty hearing in noise, but she acknowledged an improvement when using her hearing devices.

References

[1] Tillman TW, Carhart R. An expanded test for speech discrimination utilizing CNC monosyllabic words: Northwestern University auditory test no. 6 (USAF School of Aerospace Medicine Report No. SAM-TR-66–55). In: Chaiklin JB, Ventry IM, Dixon RF, eds. Hearing measurement: A book of readings. 2nd ed. Reading, MA: Addison-Wesley; 1966:226–235

[2] Walker G, Dillon H, Byrne D. Sound field audiometry: recommended stimuli and procedures. Ear Hear. 1984; 5(1): 13–21

[3] Moore K, Violetto D. FRESH noise: a fresh approach to pediatric testing. AudiologyOnline; 2016: Article 17035. www.audiologyonline.com

[4] Mancini PC, Tyler RS, Jun HJ, et al. Reliability of the minimum masking level as outcome variable in tinnitus clinical research. Am J Audiol. 2020; 29(3):429–435

[5] Sherlock LP, Formby C. Estimates of loudness, loudness discomfort, and the auditory dynamic range: normative estimates, comparison of procedures, and test-retest reliability. J Am Acad Audiol. 2005; 16(2):85–100

[6] Armstrong-Jones R. Snapping of the brain. Lancet. 1920; 196 (5066):720

[7] Pearce JM. Exploding head syndrome. Lancet. 1988; 2(8605): 270–271

[8] Ceriani CEJ, Nahas SJ. Exploding head syndrome: a review. Curr Pain Headache Rep. 2018; 22(10):63

[9] Thompson EC, Krizman J, White-Schwoch T, Nicol T, LaBella CR, Kraus N. Difficulty hearing in noise: a sequela of concussion in children. Brain Inj. 2018; 32(6):763–769

[10] Meikle, MB, Henry, JA, Griest, SE, et al. The tinnitus functional index: development of a new clinical measure for chronic, intrusive tinnitus. Ear and hearing. 2021;33(2), 153–176

[11] Jastreboff PJ. 25 years of tinnitus retraining therapy. HNO. 2015; 63(4):307–311

[12] Jastreboff PJ, Jastreboff MM. Tinnitus Retraining Therapy (TRT) as a method for treatment of tinnitus and hyperacusis patients. J Am Acad Audiol. 2000; 11(3):162–177

[13] Newman CW, Jacobson GP, Spitzer JB. Development of the tinnitus handicap inventory. Arch Otolaryngol Head Neck Surg. 1996; 122(2):143–148

[14] Khalfa S, Dubal S, Veuillet E, Perez-Diaz F, Jouvent R, Collet L. Psychometric normalization of a hyperacusis questionnaire. ORL J Otorhinolaryngol Relat Spec. 2002; 64(6):436–442

11 Tonic Tensor Tympanic Syndrome

Erin Benear

11.1 Clinical History and Description

AH, a 23-year-old male college student was seen at a private practice speech and hearing center with the chief complaint of bilateral tinnitus, describing the right to be considerably worse. Case history included subjective report and the administration of the Tinnitus Reaction Questionnaire (TRQ). Subjective report indicated that a few months prior to the appointment, he had been on a hunting trip with his grandfather. He reported the use of hearing protection devices throughout the trip. He reported that he had been on many prior hunting trips and experienced tinnitus in both ears, which he described as lasting only a few hours. After this most recent trip, his tinnitus lasted longer than usual. He denied otalgia associated with the tinnitus; however, he experienced increased anxiety due to the persistent tinnitus. The morning after his return from the trip, he reported that, upon waking, his left ear tinnitus abated, but the tinnitus in his right ear was worse than the day before. In addition to increased tinnitus, he described additional symptoms including aural pressure and sound sensitivity, in his right ear. He reported minimal dull otalgia, mild dizziness/off-steadiness and light-headedness that he associated with nausea. After a week of distressing symptoms and increased anxiety, AH was seen at an urgent care facility. He was prescribed antibiotics and steroids. A steroid shot was also administered at this appointment. AH denied any decrease in symptoms over the next 2 weeks. He reported he became increasingly more aware of his symptoms, his anxiety, and his feelings of depression. With the increased anxiety and depression, he admitted that he no longer wanted to return to school for the spring semester. He was evaluated by two different ear, nose, and throat (ENT) physicians, both of whom indicated no anatomical abnormalities. A magnetic resonance imaging (MRI) evaluation was ordered by his physician and no abnormalities were identified. Over the course of a few months, AH's symptoms increased in severity and he also began to report a significant "fluttering" in his right ear. This new symptom was causing his anxiety and depression to increase. He was seen by his ENT for follow-up and was diagnosed with tonic tensor tympanic syndrome. He reported that this diagnosis increased his anxiety substantially.

11.2 Audiological Testing

Multiple audiologic evaluations were completed prior to AH being seen in our private practice, all of which indicated hearing sensitivity within normal limits. Our evaluation began with otoscopy that revealed clear ear canals, bilaterally. Pure-tone testing at this evaluation indicated normal hearing sensitivity from 250 to 8,000 Hz bilaterally (see ▶ Fig. 11.1). The pure-tone average (PTA) was 13 dB HL for the right ear and 12 dB HL for the left ear. Tympanometry revealed type A tympanograms, bilaterally. Acoustic reflex thresholds (ARTs) were normal in both the ipsilateral and contralateral conditions for both ears. The speech recognition thresholds (SRTs) of 10 dB HL for the right ear and 15 dB HL for the left ear were consistent with the PTA of each ear. Word recognition scores, in quiet, were excellent with recorded stimuli presented at a normal conversational level of 55 dB HL. The QuickSIN, words in noise test, was administered at a presentation level of 60 dBA and revealed a 2-dB signal-to-noise ratio loss, which is a normal finding.

11.3 Questions for the Reader

1. What is Tonic Tensor Tympanic Syndrome and is it important in this case?
2. Are anxiety and depression often comorbidities in patients experiencing tinnitus?

11.4 Discussion of Questions for the Reader

1. *What is Tonic Tensor Tympanic Syndrome and is it important in this case?*
   Westcott et al describe Tonic Tensor Tympanic Syndrome (TTTS) as an involuntary, anxiety-based condition resulting in a reduced reflex threshold for the tensor tympani muscle, resulting in frequent myoclonus or spasm.[1] This often triggers additional otologic symptoms including tympanic membrane

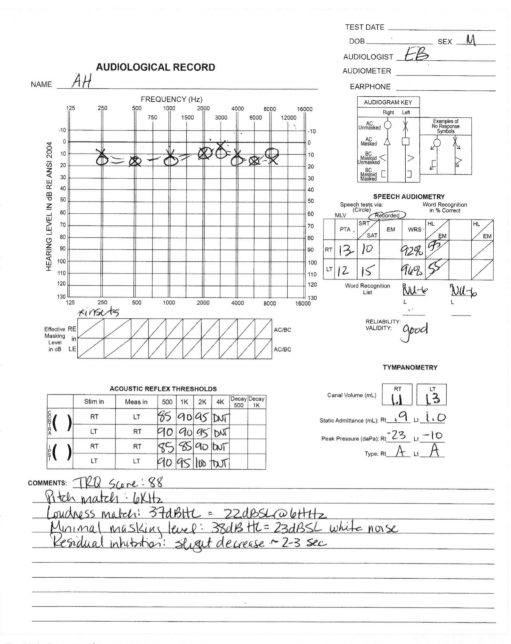

Fig. 11.1 Current audiogram.

tension and variation in middle ear ventilation. In some cases, the trigeminal nerve can become irritated resulting in central pain sensitization.[1] TTTS is often associated with an acoustic shock (AS) or a sudden, unexpected overexposure to sound that produces durable discomfort.

2. *Are anxiety and depression often comorbidities in patients experiencing tinnitus?*
Throughout the research, it is noted that TTTS symptoms are subjective and often contribute to increased levels of anxiety. Therefore, the presence of TTTS plays an important role in this case. It is noted throughout the research,

individuals with tinnitus often have psychological comorbidities. Many studies, including the study by Zöger and colleagues, have also shown individuals with tinnitus tend to have a higher prevalence of anxiety and depression compared to the general population.[2] AH noted anxiety and depression throughout his case history in addition to pain and other symptoms associated with TTTS.

11.5 Tinnitus Evaluation

Unfortunately, ultra-high-frequency audiometry could not be performed due to clinic restrictions. However, pitch match, loudness match, minimum masking level, and residual inhibition tests were conducted. The Tinnitus Reaction Questionnaire (TRQ) was also administered (▶ Fig. 11.2). Per clinic protocol, all tinnitus testing was conducted

Tinnitus Reaction Questionnaire

Patient Name __A H_____ Date_____

This questionnaire is designed to find out what sort of effects tinnitus has had on your lifestyle, general well-being, etc. Some of the effects below may apply to you, some may not. Please answer **all** questions by circling the number that best reflects how your tinnitus has affected you **over the past week.**

	Not at all	A little of the time	Some of the time	A good deal of the time	Almost all of the time
1. My tinnitus has made me unhappy.	0	1	2	3	(4)
2. My tinnitus has made me feel tense.	0	1	2	3	(4)
3. My tinnitus has made me feel irritable.	0	1	2	3	(4)
4. My tinnitus has made me feel angry.	0	1	2	(3)	4
5. My tinnitus has led me to cry.	0	(1)	2	3	4
6. My tinnitus has led me to avoid quiet situations.	0	1	2	3	(4)
7. My tinnitus has made me feel less interested in going out.	0	1	2	3	(4)
8. My tinnitus has made me feel depressed.	0	1	2	3	(4)
9. My tinnitus has made me feel annoyed.	0	1	2	3	(4)
10. My tinnitus has made me feel confused.	0	1	2	3	(4)
11. My tinnitus has "driven me crazy."	0	1	2	3	(4)
12. My tinnitus has interfered with my enjoyment of life.	0	1	2	3	(4)
13. My tinnitus has made it hard for me to concentrate.	0	1	2	(3)	4
14. My tinnitus has made it hard for me to relax.	0	1	2	3	(4)
15. My tinnitus has made me feel distressed.	0	1	2	3	(4)
16. My tinnitus has made me feel helpless.	0	1	2	3	(4)
17. My tinnitus has made me feel frustrated with things.	0	1	2	3	(4)
18. My tinnitus has interfered with my ability to work.	0	1	2	3	(4)
19. My tinnitus has led me to despair.	0	1	2	3	(4)
20. My tinnitus has led me to avoid noisy situations.	0	(1)	2	3	4
21. My tinnitus has led me to avoid social situations.	0	1	(2)	3	4
22. My tinnitus has made me feel hopeless about the future.	0	1	2	3	(4)
23. My tinnitus has interfered with my sleep.	0	1	2	(3)	4
24. My tinnitus has led me to think about suicide.	(0)	1	2	3	4
25. My tinnitus has made me feel panicky.	0	1	2	3	(4)
26. My tinnitus has made me feel tormented.	0	1	2	(3)	4
Totals:	0	2	2	12	72

Tinnitus Reaction
Based on Combined Total:

(From Wilson et al. 1991)

☐ Grade 1 – Slight (0-16)
☐ Grade 2 – Mild (18-36)
☐ Grade 3 – Moderate (38-56)
☐ Grade 4 – Severe (58-76)
☒ Grade 5 – Catastrophic (78-100)

COMBINED TOTAL:
(Add totals above)   88

V:02.08.2019

Fig. 11.2 Tinnitus reaction questionnaire.

in the ear with the most bothersome tinnitus, which for AH, was his right ear. It should be noted this clinical protocol is not a typical representation of protocols throughout the literature. The literature more often supports testing the less bothersome ear for pitch and loudness match. Variation in results could be possible if the more supported protocol had been followed.

a) Tinnitus evaluation revealed the following: pitch match (6,000 Hz), loudness match (22 dB SL re: pure-tone threshold at 6,000 Hz for the right ear), minimum masking level for white noise (23 dB SL re: white noise threshold for the right ear), and partial residual inhibition (reported decrease in volume of tinnitus for a few seconds).

b) The TRQ was administered and scored prior to oral case history. Scoring of the TRQ indicated a score of 88 (88 out of 104). The score of 88 placed the patient in the subgroup of a Grade 5 tinnitus reaction, consistent with a catastrophic reaction to his tinnitus.

11.6 Additional Questions for the Reader

1. What additional test(s) and/or questionnaires should be considered?
2. What resources should be on hand and should be utilized for this patient?

11.7 Discussion of Additional Questions for the Reader

1. *What additional test(s) and/or questionnaires should be considered?*
   a) The evaluation of ultra-high-frequency thresholds would be beneficial for additional information. Ultra-high-frequency testing could be useful, in conjunction with a traditional comprehensive diagnostic evaluation. The information gathered from ultra-high-frequency testing could assist in the counseling process, especially when explaining the cause and/or development of tinnitus. This would be especially beneficial for the patients with normal threshold throughout the traditional comprehensive audiogram as the use of ultra-high-frequency testing can evaluate the entire audibility range of human capability. As we know, patients experiencing tinnitus often need extensive counseling to facilitate learning to cope with their tinnitus.

   b) Testing the patient's loudness discomfort level (LDL) could provide additional information, specifically relating to his report of sound sensitivity.

   c) According to Kimball and colleagues, many other studies elaborate on the importance of psychological screening tools to assess the need to further evaluate a patient's mental health status.[3] Administering a depression and/or anxiety questionnaire could be extremely beneficial for this patient. The Patient Health Questionnaire (PHQ-9) is a multipurpose tool to help in screening, diagnosing, monitoring, and measuring the severity of depression. The questionnaire comes with a scoring table along with proposed treatment actions, including when to refer patient to additional professionals, such as a mental health specialist. The Generalized Anxiety Disorder 7-item (GAD-7) is a screening tool to help evaluate the possibility of a generalized anxiety disorder. This too has a scoring table that indicates severity of anxiety, ranking minimal to severe.

   d) Tinnitus Handicap Inventory (THI) and/or the Tinnitus Functional Index (TFI) are also used often as means to measure subjective burden a patient is experiencing in relation to his/her tinnitus. The THI is a tool used to evaluate the disabling consequences of tinnitus. The THI can also be used later, after treatment, to measure outcomes. The TFI has eight subscales of measurement, looking at the patient's sense of control, the intrusiveness of the tinnitus, cognitive interference, disturbances in sleep, auditory concerns, and issues with relaxation, emotional distress, and overall quality of life. Both questionnaires are regularly utilized in the clinical setting and would have provided additional information on the patient's personal reaction to tinnitus.

2. *What resources should be on hand and should be utilized for this patient?*
   a) It is always important to know your state and national agencies and resources. This patient could benefit from support groups and other forms of therapeutic release, not only for tinnitus but also for his anxiety and depression.

b) Having specific contact information for multiple professionals is vital when dealing with patients who might need help beyond audiology. Patients often need to be referred to psychologists or psychiatrists to help manage their anxiety and depression.

11.8 Final Diagnosis and Recommended Treatment

AH's evaluation revealed thresholds within normal limits at all frequencies tested, normal immittance testing, both tympanometry and acoustic reflexes, and severe unilateral tinnitus. AH's most significant symptoms included his anxiety and depression that had begun to affect his daily life. The mental health conditions were attributed, at least in part, to his tinnitus severity and the diagnosis of TTTS. Addressing his anxiety and depression was of most importance for this patient. He was provided with the contact information of a local registered therapist who specialized in anxiety, emotional disturbance, and behavioral issues. Ultra-high-frequency audiometry was recommended for additional information and possible etiopathogenesis. In regard to his tinnitus, sound therapy was recommended with a smartphone app or sound generator. On ear devices were discussed; however, AH requested the least invasive approach first. As we know, sound therapy is also a treatment option for patients with hyperacusis, and Westcott's research suggests that an effective hyperacusis treatment reduces the frequency and severity of TTTS symptoms.[1] AH was counseled on the results of his hearing tests and he received extensive counseling on the mechanisms of tinnitus, common causes and treatments, and additional information on TTTS.

11.9 Outcome

Case history, diagnostic evaluation, and counseling required a 2-hour appointment. After extensive counseling, AH reported a decrease in anxiety about his condition. He indicated no other professional had taken the extra time to explain his diagnosis. He reported, due to the lack of information provided by his previous professionals, he and his girlfriend were researching information online (through uncited sources). This flood of information reportedly increased his anxiety. He acknowledged that activity during the lengthy appointment increased understanding about his condition and he expressed the desire to follow-up with a mental health professional. He reported he was going to utilize a sound generator while at home. He also reported he felt he would be able to return to school with some relief. He reported he would return with any new symptoms or concerns.

11.10 Clinician Self-Efficacy

- Patients with tinnitus, hyperacusis, and other sound sensitivities often also experience anxiety and depression. This has to be considered when providing care and information to your patient.
- Counseling deficits can lead to additional questions and increased concern for our patients.[4]
- Emphasizing patient-centered care in our counseling practices could improve patients' perception of their diagnosis.

References

[1] Westcott M, Sanchez TG, Diges I, et al. Tonic tensor tympani syndrome in tinnitus and hyperacusis patients: a multi-clinic prevalence study. Noise Health. 2013; 15(63):117–128

[2] Zöger S, Svedlund J, Holgers KM. Relationship between tinnitus severity and psychiatric disorders. Psychosomatics. 2006; 47(4):282–288

[3] Kimball SH, Hamilton T, Benear E, Baldwin J. Determining emotional tone and verbal behavior in patients with tinnitus and hyperacusis: an exploratory mixed-methods study. Am J Audiol. 2019; 28(3):660–672

[4] Pearson N, Munoz K, Landon T, Corbin-Lewis K. Counseling skills in audiology. Hear J. 2019; 72:50–51

Suggested Readings

Aazh H, Moore BCJ. Factors associated with depression in patients with tinnitus and hyperacusis. Am J Audiol. 2017; 26(4):562–569

Stewart M, Brown JB, Donner A, et al. The impact of patient-centered care on outcomes. J Fam Pract. 2000; 49(9):796–804 online

Tyler RS, Pienkowski M, Roncancio ER, et al. A review of hyperacusis and future directions: part I. Definitions and manifestations. Am J Audiol. 2014; 23(4):402–419

12 Tinnitus Secondary to Barotrauma

Trevor Courouleau

12.1 Clinical History/Description

A 56-year-old female was seen for an audiologic evaluation in 2018 following the onset of pressure in the right ear and constant ringing tinnitus in the left ear during initial ascent on an airplane flight. Patient reported significant pain and subsequent discomfort for the duration of the flight that increased during final descent. She denied history of otologic infection, otorrhea, vertigo, noise exposure, or previous hearing aid use.

12.2 Audiologic Testing

Otoscopy showed clear ear canals bilaterally. Tympanic membranes appeared normal. Tympanometry revealed type A tympanograms bilaterally. Ipsilateral acoustic reflexes were absent, bilaterally. Speech recognition thresholds were within normal limits, bilaterally (right ear: 15 dB HL, left ear: 15 dB HL) (▶ Fig. 12.1). Pure-tone testing indicated a normal sloping to mild sensorineural hearing loss, bilaterally. A negative pure-tone Stenger was noted at 3,000 Hz. Word recognition was excellent, bilaterally (100% at 60 dB HL).

12.3 Additional Testing

Follow-up with an otolaryngologist (ENT) was recommended due to the patient's report and symptoms consistent with barotrauma. The patient was scheduled to repeat audiologic evaluation following medical management, and was advised that if the tinnitus persisted in the left ear, further tinnitus evaluation and management with masking would be considered.

Subsequent testing was completed 1 month later. The patient reported a tube was placed in the right ear by the ENT. The patient felt that her tinnitus had changed and was now louder in the right ear. The patient also reported increased hearing loss in her right ear, with pain. She was prescribed antibiotic drops post-tube insertion by the ENT. During an audiometric follow-up exam, otoscopy revealed a tube and debris in the right ear. The left ear was unremarkable. Tympanometry for the right ear showed a flat tympanogram with a large ear canal volume, consistent with pressure equalization (PE)

tube patency. Tympanometry for the left ear was within normal limits. Ipsilateral acoustic reflexes were absent. Speech recognition thresholds were 20 dB HL, bilaterally. Pure-tone testing for the right ear revealed a mixed hearing loss with a 20 dB HL decrease in thresholds from her prior hearing evaluation, and an air-bone gap at 250 Hz (consistent with tube placement). Pure-tone testing for the left ear showed stable sensorineural hearing loss as compared to first exam. A negative pure-tone Stenger was noted at 250 Hz. Word recognition scores were excellent, bilaterally (100% at 60 dB HL). The patient was scheduled to follow-up with her ENT in 2 weeks. Repeat audiologic testing was recommended following her ENT appointment to monitor any changes in her medical management as well as her hearing sensitivity and tinnitus (▶ Fig. 12.2).

12.4 Questions for the Reader

1. How common is barotrauma and what is the typical clinical presentation?
2. In cases of unilateral tinnitus, is it sufficient to provide masking only to the affected ear?
3. What evidence is available to share with patients in order to illustrate the notion that binaural sound enrichment is the most appropriate form of tinnitus masking?

12.5 Discussion of Questions for the Reader

1. *How common is barotrauma and what is the typical clinical presentation?*
   Barotrauma refers to injuries caused by increased air or water pressure after a flight or deep water diving, and is commonly seen in the ear. O'Neill and Frank[1] indicate that SCUBA divers, commercial divers, and patients undergoing hyperbaric oxygen treatment comprise the population most at risk for barotrauma. Patients most typically report pain and pressure accompanied by varying degrees of hearing loss. Tympanic membrane rupture accompanied by blood in the ear canal and middle ear is often a result of barotrauma.
2. *In cases of unilateral tinnitus, is it sufficient to provide masking only to the affected ear?*

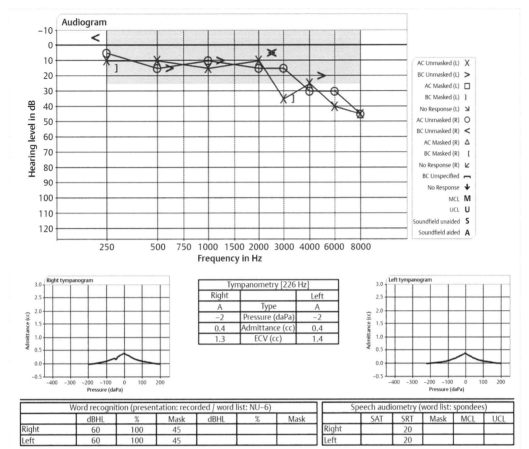

Fig. 12.1 Initial evaluation.

Many patients with unilateral tinnitus may be under the impression that masking, or aiding the affected ear only, is an appropriate course of action. While unilateral masking makes intuitive sense, it neglects to consider that the central auditory pathway contains numerous sites for binaural interaction of nerve impulses and their processing sites. It is likely that the neural event that produces tinnitus appearing unilaterally, in fact, occupies both channels of the auditory pathway, and is merely more powerful on one side. Masking the perception on the stronger side has the potential to "unmask" the perception contralaterally, thereby increasing awareness of tinnitus in the "unaffected" ear. To minimize the likelihood of such an experience for the patient, binaural masking/sound enrichment is indicated in all cases.

3. *What evidence is available to share with patients in order to illustrate the notion that binaural sound enrichment is the most appropriate form of tinnitus masking?*

Evidence to support the binaural provision of noise may be observed most readily during measures of minimum masking level. If tinnitus were produced in the ear, then it would be susceptible to masking in a manner similar to a pure-tone stimulus in a routine audiometric

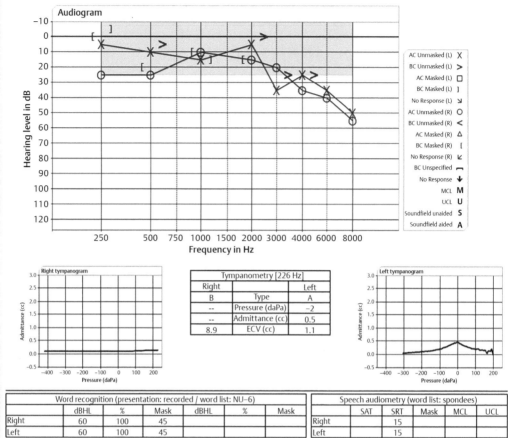

Fig. 12.2 Follow-up evaluation.

evaluation. In order to mask a right-sided tinnitus with a masker presented to the left ear, the masker level would need to overcome interaural attenuation (IA) in order to mask. Numerous investigators demonstrated something different; the amount of energy needed to mask the "unaffected" ear is typically in the order of 5 to 15 dB SL re: the masker level required in the tinnitus ear. Such values fall far below the typical IA values of 40 to 60 dB required to mask an externally generated tone. In other words, tinnitus does not behave as an external tone, as its masking does not require compensation for IA.

12.6 Final Diagnosis and Recommended Treatment

The patient was seen approximately 6 months later. She reported hearing a low-frequency narrowband tinnitus noise in the right ear and cicadas/crickets in the back of her head. She reported that her tinnitus was a 7/10 for severity and she requested any relief available. Otoscopy for the right ear revealed nonoccluding cerumen. Tympanometry for the right ear revealed a large volume flat tympanogram consistent w/ patent PE tube. A tinnitus evaluation was completed for the right ear. Pitch match was established at 500 Hz (with narrowband noise quality) at 45 dB HL. Minimum masking level was 60 dB HL using white noise. Residual inhibition was tested at 70 d HL and was found to be present, but very brief as the patient reported her tinnitus was gone for a "split second" and then returned. Management strategies were reviewed with the patient, including ear-level tinnitus masking devices, informational counseling, and personal adjustment counseling. The patient was advised that referrals could also be considered for cognitive behavioral therapy (CBT), biofeedback, and medication for symptoms. It was determined that the patient's tinnitus would be best managed with a masker/hearing aid ear-level devices fit binaurally. Progressive Tinnitus Management materials were uploaded to the patient's portal for self-guided informational management.[2]

The patient declined binaural masking and was fitted with a right ear receiver-in-canal hearing aid/masker in 2019. The device and tinnitus masker were enabled and set to patient preference. She reported her tinnitus in the right ear was more "mellow." However, the patient was able to hear tinnitus more in her left ear. A 2-week follow-up revealed that the patient was not doing well. She reported the locust sound was less intrusive but that she was still able to hear tinnitus in the left ear. Masker settings were adjusted to patient preference.

12.7 Outcome

At her most recent appointment in 2019, the patient reported her masker was too loud. Amplification was turned off and masker settings were extensively changed for patient comfort. A trial/demo hearing aid was fitted on the left ear with a tinnitus masker (in addition to using the device already fitted on the right ear). Initial findings in clinic were positive, with the patient reporting her tinnitus seemed completely "dulled out."

12.8 Self-Efficacy for the Clinician

- Patients should be counseled on the basics of binaural sound processing, and therefore should be encouraged to utilize tinnitus sound therapy in both ears.

Acknowledgment

This material is the result of work supported with resources and the use of facilities at the OSU Speech-Language-Hearing Clinic.

References

[1] ONeill OJ, Frank AJ. Ear barotrauma. [Updated 2019 Dec 20]. In: StatPearls [Internet]. Treasure Island (FL): StatPearls Publishing; 2020. https://www.ncbi.nlm.nih.gov/books/NBK499851/

[2] Henry JA, Zaug TL, Myers PJ, Kendall CJ. How to manage your tinnitus: a step-by-step workbook. 3rd ed. VA RR&D National Center for Rehabilitative Auditory Research (NCRAR); 2019

13 Acoustic Shock Disorder

Marc Fagelson

13.1 Background

Mr. H, a 65-year-old male, was evaluated in 2012, about 4 months after he experienced a stressful event that involved high sound levels. As a consequence of the event, the patient noticed extreme discomfort in the presence of sounds that were once tolerable. In addition, his preexisting tinnitus worsened immediately and durably following the event. The patient's sound exposure history covered more than 35 years of occupational and military-related noise exposure. The patient denied familial history of hearing loss and vertigo. He expressed no health concerns other than hypertension that predated the sound exposure. The patient was diagnosed subsequently with depression and anxiety. He denied nicotine, ethanol, and recreational drug use, and reported infrequent use of over-the-counter medication for sleep.

The patient was offered the opportunity to disclose the nature of the auditory event with which he associated tinnitus exacerbation and sound intolerance. His narrative centered on exposure to the horn of a firetruck—at a distance of less than 50 meters and directed at his right ear—from the front yard of his home. While he was accustomed to the sound of the horn, due to his home's proximity to the firehouse, in this instance, he jumped at the sound in a manner noticeable to the driver of the truck. In the patient's recounting, the driver *deliberately and unnecessarily* deployed the horn repeatedly after observing the patient startle. Immediately he felt sharp pain in the right ear and his tinnitus grew louder, a change consistent with reactive tinnitus. Since that exposure, the patient observed pain in the right ear in response

to a variety of sounds, in particular high-pitched and impulsive sounds. The patient reported avoiding places he expected to be loud, and he experienced anxiety when considering the possibility of painful reactions to sound. This combination of pain, anxiety, tinnitus, and sound intolerance was specified by Westcott et al[1] as a demonstration of tonic tensor tympani syndrome, perhaps resulting from acute exposures in certain occupational settings and consistent with an acoustic shock.[2]

13.2 Assessment

Pure-tone air conduction testing was completed approximately 4 years prior to the patient's encounter in the tinnitus clinic, and his tinnitus appointment occurred 4 months postexposure. His pure-tone thresholds, both prior to and following the exposure (▶ Table 13.1), revealed sloping mild-to-moderate severe hearing loss that worsened by 10 to 20 dB HL at 3, 4, 6, and 8 kHz in the right ear. Pure-tone thresholds decreased similarly in the left ear, although it should be noted that the patient had slightly better hearing in the left ear prior to and following the exposure. Middle ear measures and acoustic reflex findings prior to the exposure were consistent with sensorineural hearing loss. The Tinnitus Functional Index (TFI)[3] and Tinnitus Handicap Inventory (THI)[4] were administered. The patient's scores of 70/100 on the THI and 86/100 on the TFI (all eight domains averaged > 7/10) were in the most severe categories for each instrument. The patient rated both his tinnitus severity and sound intolerance at 9/10; however, he asserted that his

Table 13.1 Pure-tone thresholds in dB HL before (pre-PT) and after (post-PT) sudden hearing loss onset related to acoustic shock event

	250 Hz	500 Hz	1000 Hz	1500 Hz	2000 Hz	3000 Hz	4000 Hz	8000 Hz
Pre-PT R	10	20	20		30	45	60	70
Post-PT R	20	20	20	25	45	55	75	90
Pre-PT L	20	10	15		15	30	45	55
Post-PT L	15	20	15		30	50	65	80
AR RI		100	85		85			
AR RC		105	NR		NR			
AR LI		100	85		90			
AR LC		90	95		95			

aversion to many routinely experienced sounds was more substantial than his tinnitus distress.

13.3 Questions for the Reader

1. What are the elements of a case history that suggest an acoustic shock?
2. Are there intake forms other than those employed by audiologists that would be of value for a patient who had experienced an acoustic shock?
3. What distinguishes a patient suffering from an acoustic shock from other forms of sound intolerance?

13.4 Discussion of Questions for the Reader

1. *What are the elements of a case history that suggest an acoustic shock?*
   Patients who endure an acoustic shock may report tinnitus, fullness, and change in hearing, sound intolerance, and in particular, sound-associated pain. Many patients can recall a specific event after which the symptoms started; hence, asking a patient about the onset event should be an element of the case history. Oftentimes the specific event was associated with employment, resulting in the sense that the patient's workplace is no longer safe.
2. *Are there intake forms other than those employed by audiologists that would be of value for a patient who had experienced an acoustic shock?*
   If the patient complains of tinnitus, then several intake forms may be employed—the TFI and THI at a minimum. Because acoustic shock disorder (ASD) often features substantial emotional and mental health complications, clinicians may find that administration of the Hospital Anxiety-Depression Screener (HADS)[5] would indicate the need for a mental health referral. With regard to sound insensitivity, the Inventory of Hyperacusis Symptoms (IHS)[6] can provide information regarding challenging sounds, environments, and opportunities to support counseling and rehabilitation efforts.
3. *What distinguishes a patient suffering from an acoustic shock from other forms of sound intolerance?*
   The primary differences relate to the patient's complaints of sharp pain in the ear accompanying sound levels that others find tolerable. The report of pain is also emphasized by Westcott et al[1] and McFerran.[2] In addition, patients with ASD often have normal thresholds in spite of their reports regarding sounds appearing dull, ears feeling full, and tinnitus that appears to worsen in response to many environmental sounds.

13.5 Outcome

The patient was provided a set of hearing aids that contained rudimentary tinnitus masking options. Device default setting included a low-level masking noise to accompany the hearing aid settings. He returned to the clinic 6 months later at which time the TFI and THI revealed decreases in scores from 86/100 to 57/100 on the TFI, and from 70/100 to 44/100 on the THI, both clinically significant decreases from initial administration. Despite these improvements, the patient reported that many environmental sounds remained too loud, and that pain was routinely produced by sounds that did not bother other people, particularly high-pitched sounds, horns, and sirens.

13.6 Clinician Self-Efficacy

The approach to patient management centered on desensitization, and encouragement to minimize sound avoidance. Hearing aid use was intended as an element of increasing exposure to sound, as was the need to minimize avoidance of challenging situations. Although the patient in general concurred with these strategies, he cautioned against clinicians vigorously encouraging patients to practice exposure. He reported a number of occasions during which, with good intentions, he attended an event at which he anticipated high-level sounds. When exposed to the sounds, he reportedly felt pain. He tempered the desire to withdraw with the well-intended counseling and suggestions from the health care provider. Subsequent to some attempts to participate in noisy events, he observed a temporary exacerbation of symptoms, or a set back. As a result, the patient had to learn on his own to navigate not just environmental exposures, but the need to maintain sound enrichment without triggering a setback. In his words, the difference is that his recognition of symptom sources, mechanisms, and potential exacerbators facilitates their management.

13.7 What Evidence Is There to Support Desensitization Strategies?

Desensitization strategies are ubiquitous, and address many diverse aspects of life. A brief sampling of desensitization targets—anxiety, pain, medication management, working with a child, or a pet, to modify behavior—reinforces our own anecdotal observations that thoughts and behaviors can be modified by exposures to a variety of environmental and sensory events. The phenomenon of the "acquired taste" often includes an element of desensitization. Service dogs are trained to tolerate all manner of distractions and strangers, while others, such as those who will hunt, could be trained to respond vigorously to a small inventory of stimuli. With regard to hearing and sound intolerance, Formby and colleagues[7] demonstrated the rapidity with which the sensation of loudness could be modified over a few weeks. Participants used for 2 to 4 weeks either low-level masking noise or earplugs; those who wore maskers experienced an increase in loudness tolerance (i.e., they could tolerate higher levels of sound than prior to using the maskers), and those who used earplugs experienced the opposite, a decrease in sound levels tolerated. Although desensitization risks overstimulation and the potential for setbacks, the strategy remains an important element supporting management and rehabilitation of sound-induced discomfort.

References

[1] Westcott M, Sanchez TG, Diges I, et al. Tonic tensor tympani syndrome in tinnitus and hyperacusis patients: a multi-clinic prevalence study. Noise Health. 2013; 15(63):117–128

[2] McFerran D. Acoustic shock. In: Baguley DM, Fagelson M, eds. Tinnitus: clinical and research perspectives. San Diego, CA: Plural Publishing; 2015:197–212

[3] Meikle MB, Henry JA, Griest SE, et al. The tinnitus functional index: development of a new clinical measure for chronic, intrusive tinnitus. Ear Hear. 2012; 33(2):153–176

[4] Newman CW, Jacobson GP, Spitzer JB. Development of the Tinnitus Handicap Inventory. Arch Otolaryngol Head Neck Surg. 1996; 122(2):143–148

[5] Zigmond AS, Snaith RP. The hospital anxiety and depression scale. Acta Psychiatr Scand. 1983; 67(6):361–370

[6] Greenberg B, Carlos M. Psychometric properties and factor structure of a new scale to measure hyperacusis: introducing the inventory of hyperacusis symptoms. Ear Hear. 2018; 39 (5):1025–1034

[7] Formby C, Sherlock LP, Gold SL. Adaptive plasticity of loudness induced by chronic attenuation and enhancement of the acoustic background. J Acoust Soc Am. 200 3; 114(1): 55–58

14 Acoustic Shock

Don McFerran

14.1 Clinical History

A 37-year-old woman (KD) presented at the Accident and Emergency department of our hospital. She reported that she worked for a local health care facility in which patients with minor medical conditions were assessed and managed. During the daytime, the center was open to the public but after 10 p.m. the doors were closed and only patients with prearranged appointments were admitted. Part of her duties involved using the out-of-hours intercom system to admit such patients. Two days previously she had been at work at approximately 10:30 when the intercom had buzzed. She picked up the intercom's telephone handset to her right ear and established that the female patient using the intercom did not have an appointment. She explained to the patient that the center was closed to walk-in patients and that she would need to go to the main District General Hospital for assessment and treatment. The patient then suddenly screamed loudly into the intercom and unleashed a tirade of verbal abuse. KD reported sudden pain in the right ear, a sensation as if her head were about to explode and severe distress. She described the pain as a physical pain, not a sound-related phenomenon. She felt that the hearing was muffled and she had a sensation of blockage of the right ear. There was, however, no sustained tinnitus or vertigo. She reported that she had become extremely sensitive to sound since the time of the incident. Initial examination was normal.

14.2 Audiological Testing

Pure-tone audiometry showed normal hearing thresholds in the range 250 Hz to 8 kHz (▶ Fig. 14.1). Tympanometry showed normal type A tympanograms bilaterally (▶ Fig. 14.2). No other testing was performed at this stage. The medical team explained that examination was normal and there was no evidence of significant acoustic trauma. She was given reassurance and advised that her symptoms would probably settle spontaneously but if this failed to happen, then she should contact her General Practitioner.

A month after the exposure, she still had unpleasant symptoms and after a consultation with her General Practitioner she was referred to our tinnitus clinic.

14.3 Questions for the Reader

1. What additional case history information might be useful?
2. What additional audiological testing could be considered?

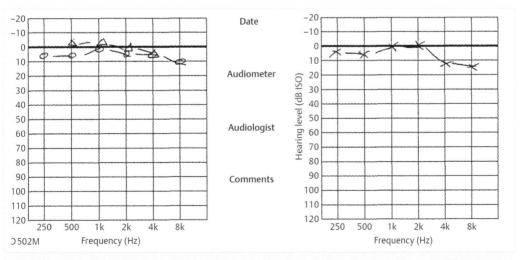

Fig. 14.1 Initial air conduction (AC) and unmasked bone conduction (BC) pure-tone audiogram, demonstrating normal hearing.

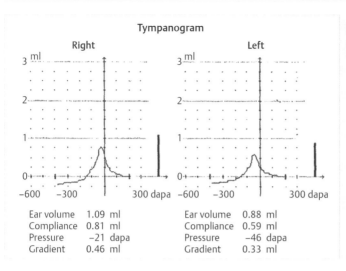

Fig. 14.2 Initial tympanogram, demonstrating normal type A tympanograms bilaterally.

3. What are the pros and cons of additional audiological testing?
4. What other assessment tools could be employed?
5. What is acoustic shock syndrome?

14.4 Discussion of Questions for the Reader

1. *What additional case history information might be useful?*
   It would be useful to explore the sound sensitivity symptoms in more depth, both to categorize her impaired sound tolerance and to assess its impact on her activities of daily living. Specific areas to investigate would include the impact, if any, on her sleep and concentration, the impact on family life, and the impact on her ability to work. It would also be relevant to ask about her past medical history, particularly those areas related to stress and anxiety.

2. *What additional audiological testing could be considered?*
   Tests for hidden hearing loss such as extended range audiometry, otoacoustic emissions and click-evoked electrocochleography[10,2] could be considered to determine whether she had sustained auditory damage that had not been picked up by conventional pure-tone audiometry. Loudness discomfort level (LDL) testing could be undertaken to assess her sound sensitivity issues. Acoustic reflex testing could be performed as a general measure of auditory function.

3. *What are the pros and cons of additional audiological testing?*
   Hidden hearing loss tests could give some more diagnostic information, but such tests are time consuming to perform and would not alter the subsequent management. Performing LDL testing in a patient who complains of impaired sound tolerance is a very contentious topic: the tests can help diagnostically but involve exposing a sound-sensitive patient to a potentially noxious stimulus. Acoustic reflex testing can give useful information about the entire auditory pathway but involves exposing the patient to high sound levels during the test. None of these tests are crucial to reach a diagnosis and plan treatment.

4. *What other assessment tools could be employed?*
   There are multiple health care questionnaires for assessing such patients, including questionnaires for tinnitus, hyperacusis, sleep disturbance, and mental health.

5. *What is acoustic shock syndrome?*
   Acoustic shock is a group of symptoms arising in individuals who have been exposed to sudden unexpected sound.[3,4,5] The causative sounds are not necessarily dangerously loud but do have a very short rise time. The condition was initially reported in call center staff in Denmark and Australia who had received an unexpected sound through their telecommunications headsets or handsets.[3,6] As clinicians have become more familiar with the condition, cases have been reported where the noise did not originate from telecommunications equipment. Common

symptoms include pain in or around the ear, tinnitus, dizziness, aural fullness, impaired sound tolerance, headaches, sleep disturbance, hypervigilance, and psychological distress. Various pathophysiological mechanisms for acoustic shock have been suggested, including tonic tensor tympani syndrome,[5,7,8] but this remains speculative and the exact cause remains obscure. Acoustic shock has not been universally accepted by health care professionals and many remain skeptical of its existence. Some clinicians, particularly those who are involved in medicolegal practice feel that the symptoms are partly or entirely psychological.[6,9,10]

14.5 Additional Clinical History and Testing

KD's health prior to this event had been excellent: her only significant past medical history was of hypothyroidism, well controlled by treatment with thyroxine. Questioning regarding her recent medical history revealed that her sleep had been severely affected in the period immediately after the sound exposure. She experienced problems both with delayed onset of sleep and with early wakening, although this had improved by the time she was seen in the tinnitus clinic. She reported that she was generally able to tolerate everyday sounds, although sudden noise from her children

caused pain at times and she found traffic noise unpleasant. She was able to visit a supermarket and attend a jazz exercise class without problem. She was, however, extremely anxious about using telephones at home and especially in her workplace, describing symptoms suggestive of panic attacks. Her fear of telephones was making it extremely difficult for her to perform her workplace duties. We had a long conversation with KD and explained the further options. We explained that it was not essential to perform any further testing but one of her ongoing issues was that she felt that she was being disbelieved by her family, employer, and health care professionals, and was therefore very keen to obtain some kind of proof of her condition. After considerable explanation we proceeded with pure-tone LDL testing at frequencies 500, 1,000, 2,000, and 4,000 Hz, although we deviated from standard protocol and started the test at her hearing threshold rather than a higher level. The test confirmed abnormal LDLs, worse on the affected right side (▶ Fig. 14.3): mean LDL on the right side was 73.75 dB (range 70–80 dB) and on the left side mean LDL was 86.25 (range 80–95 dB) (normal LDLs for people with normal hearing should be 95 dB or greater[11]). We considered the use of questionnaires, but she did not complain of tinnitus and her sleep problem had largely resolved spontaneously. There was no English language validated hyperacusis questionnaire (HQ) at this time: Khalfa's HQ was published in 2002 in an English language journal but the validation study

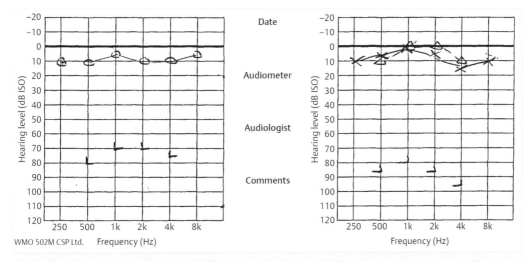

Fig. 14.3 Follow-up pure-tone audiogram with loudness discomfort levels (LDLs), demonstrating abnormal LDLs, worse on the right side.

was undertaken using the original French version of the questionnaire on a French speaking population.[12] It was not until 2015 that the HQ underwent an English validation exercise.[13] She had seen her workplace Occupational Health team and they had arranged for her to see a clinical psychologist. A mental health questionnaire was therefore deemed unnecessary.

14.6 Additional Question for the Reader

1. What treatment options are available for acoustic shock?

14.7 Discussion of Additional Question for the Reader

1. *What treatment options are available for acoustic shock?*

   There is no good evidence base regarding the treatment of acoustic shock and to a certain extent treatment has to be tailored to individual patients depending on their personal symptoms. Pain and impaired sound tolerance tend to be the most persistent symptoms in this patient cohort.[7] Counseling and sound therapy are frequently used but care must be taken with sound therapy as many of the patients—including KD in this case—have phonophobia and hypervigilance.[4] The input of physical therapists and pain specialists may be helpful for persistent pain symptoms. Stress management and, if necessary, formal psychological help may be required. If insomnia is an issue, sleep hygiene measures or referral to a sleep clinic may be appropriate.

14.8 Final Diagnosis and Recommended Treatment

We confirmed a diagnosis of acoustic shock: KD was very relieved to have this formal diagnosis. We arranged counseling, relaxation training, and sound therapy using environmental sound rather than ear level sound generators.

14.9 Outcome

Most of her symptoms settled, although she continued to find being in her workplace very problematic. Eventually she decided to leave this employment and set up her own photography business, fulfilling a long-held dream.

References

[1] Vinodh RS, Veeranna N. Evaluation of acoustic shock induced early hearing loss with audiometer and distortion product otoacoustic emissions. Indian J Med Sci. 2010; 64(3):132–139

[2] Liberman MC, Epstein MJ, Cleveland SS, Wang H, Maison SF. Toward a differential diagnosis of hidden hearing loss in humans. PLoS One. 2016; 11(9):e0162726

[3] Milhinch JC. Acoustic shock injury: real or imaginary. AudiologyOnline; 2002. Retrieved August 11 2021, from http://www.audiologyonline.com/articles/acoustic-shock-injury-real-or-1172

[4] Westcott M. Acoustic shock injury (ASI). Acta Otolaryngol Suppl. 2006; 556(556):54–58

[5] McFerran DJ, Baguley DM. Acoustic shock. J Laryngol Otol. 2007; 121(4):301–305

[6] Lawton BW. Audiometric findings in call centre workers exposed to acoustic shock. Proc Inst Acoust. 2003; 25:249–258

[7] Westcott M. Acoustic shock disorder. In: Proceedings of "Tinnitus Discovery": Asia-Pacific Tinnitus Symposium, 11–12 September 2009, Auckland, New Zealand. NZMJ 2010;123(1311):25–31

[8] Westcott M, Sanchez TG, Diges I, et al. Tonic tensor tympani syndrome in tinnitus and hyperacusis patients: a multi-clinic prevalence study. Noise Health. 2013; 15(63):117–128

[9] Parker W, Parker V, Parker G, Parker A. "Acoustic shock": a new occupational disease? Observations from clinical and medico-legal practice. Int J Audiol. 2014; 53(10):764–769

[10] Hooper RE. Acoustic shock controversies. J Laryngol Otol. 2014; 128 Suppl 2:S2–S9

[11] Sherlock LP, Formby C. Estimates of loudness, loudness discomfort, and the auditory dynamic range: normative estimates, comparison of procedures, and test-retest reliability. J Am Acad Audiol. 2005; 16(2):85–100

[12] Khalfa S, Dubal S, Veuillet E, Perez-Diaz F, Jouvent R, Collet L. Psychometric normalization of a hyperacusis questionnaire. ORL J Otorhinolaryngol Relat Spec. 2002; 64(6):436–442

[13] Fackrell K, Fearnley C, Hoare DJ, Sereda M. Hyperacusis Questionnaire as a tool for measuring hypersensitivity to sound in a tinnitus research population. BioMed Res Int. 2015; 2015:290425

Suggested Reading

McFerran D. Acoustic shock, In: Baguley DM, Fagelson M, eds. Tinnitus: clinical and research perspectives. San Diego, CA: Plural Publishing; 2016:181–196

15 Pulsatile Tinnitus

Jamie Myers and Rebecca Jimenez

15.1 Clinical History and Description

WA, an 81-year-old male, was seen at an ENT office in May of 2019 for a routine audiological examination. Audiological testing revealed moderate-to-profound symmetrical sensorineural hearing loss, reportedly stable since 2013. WA is an experienced and successful hearing aid wearer, fit with in-the-ear (ITE) devices since 1995, all the same brand. His current devices were not functioning properly, and he decided to order new ITE hearing devices at this date's appointment. After the initial fit of his new hearing instruments in June 2019, the patient complained of hearing his heartbeat, a sensation of pulsatile tinnitus, in his left ear. The patient noted that he did not experience pulsatile tinnitus with his previous ITE devices. Referral to the otolaryngologist in the office for further evaluation was suggested, but the patient refused. WA admitted to recent heart issues and stents being placed, and referral back to the cardiologist was also suggested. The patient refused the referrals, stating that since he never experienced this issue with his previous hearing aids, he was convinced that it was the hearing aids causing the sensation.

Fine-tuning adjustments to the left device were made, such as decreasing low-frequency gain, overall gain, and maximum power output (MPO), but the patient continued to hear the pulsatile tinnitus in his left ear. WA wore the devices until October 2019 and when he returned, he reported ongoing pulsatile tinnitus and requested further adjustments be made to the device. At that time, new open jaw earmold impressions were made of the left ear canal and the left device was sent back to the manufacturer for remake with a larger vent. However, after the remade hearing aid was fit, the patient continued to hear the pulsatile tinnitus. In November 2019, the hearing aid manufacturer representative was called for assistance with this patient. When the manufacturer's audiologist accompanied the patient to the appointment, the patient noted that when he wedged a cotton ball between the device and the outer ear, near the triangular fossa, to push down on the device, he no longer heard his heartbeat. The left device was then sent back to the manufacturer to have the helix portion built up to recreate that effect. In January 2020, the patient returned and reported he remained aware of the pulsatile tinnitus. The manufacturer's audiologist again came to the appointment in order to assess the physical fit. The patient reiterated that he never heard his heartbeat with his previous devices, so the current devices were sent in with his previous devices to try to replicate the physical fitting of the devices that did not produce the pulsing sensation. At that time, the patient stated that he had a pacemaker placed in December of 2019. It was again recommended that the patient have an evaluation from his otolaryngologist and cardiologist. WA agreed to see his cardiologist who reported no findings that would account for the pulsatile tinnitus. The cardiologist recommended reducing the overall gain in the devices, specifically from 2,000 to 4,000 Hz; however, those specific adjustments, similar to those attempted by the audiologists, did not relieve the pulsatile tinnitus.

In September 2020, the manufacturer's audiologist returned to see the patient due to these ongoing issues. Sound therapy using white noise that was shaped to produce equal sensation level across the patient's pure-tone thresholds was attempted, but minimum masking level could not be obtained; regardless of masker spectrum or level, the tinnitus remained audible. The clinical audiologist referred the patient again to her ENT colleague. A CT angiogram and CT scan of the temporal bone were performed. The CT scans showed a dehiscence of the temporal bone portion that would normally separate the Eustachian tube from the internal carotid artery. The manufacturer's audiologist tapered the end of the ITE device with the clinic's Redwing modification drill in order to reduce contact with the ear canal, but maintain device retention. Following this modification, the patient reported relief from the pulsatile tinnitus. The audiologist called to check on the patient at 1- and 2-week intervals following this appointment and reported no further issues with left pulsatile tinnitus.

15.2 Audiological Testing

A routine audiological evaluation was performed. Otoscopy revealed clear canals, bilaterally. Tympanometry was performed and yielded Type A tympanograms, bilaterally. Pure-tone testing revealed a symmetric, moderate to profound sensorineural hearing loss. Speech recognition thresholds were 65 dB HL, bilaterally, consistent with the pure-tone average of both ears. Word recognition scores, using recorded word list in quiet at 95 dB HL, were 48% in the right ear and 64% in the left ear. The patient's hearing loss has remained stable with no clinically significant changes in his thresholds or word recognition since 2013.

15.3 Question for the Reader

1. What is pulsatile tinnitus and is it important in this case?

15.4 Discussion of Question for the Reader

1. *What is pulsatile tinnitus and is it important in this case?*
   The patient may report a pulsating sound that does not originate from an outside source and is typically in time with a person's heartbeat. Pulsatile tinnitus is the most common type of somatosensory tinnitus, or tinnitus originating from a bodily system.[1] This may be due to the proximity of the internal carotid artery and jugular artery to the middle and inner ears. Pulsatile tinnitus could be caused by a few factors such as dehiscence of surrounding bones or an arteriovenous malformation (AVM). Pulsatile tinnitus can be exacerbated by health issues such as high blood pressure, hyperthyroidism, carotid blockage, glomus tumors, and aneurisms.[2] Due to the seriousness of these conditions, it is critical for the patient to seek medical attention to ensure that his overall health is examined, and a proper diagnosis is made before providing audiologic rehabilitation that addresses this symptom.[3]

15.5 Tinnitus Evaluation

Due to the nature of the tinnitus, tinnitus pitch and loudness evaluation were not performed. Sound therapy was attempted through the hearing devices; however, the tinnitus remained audible.

15.6 Additional Question for the Reader

1. What resources should be on hand and should be utilized for this patient?

15.7 Discussion of Additional Question for the Reader

1. *What resources should be on hand and should be utilized for this patient?*
   When pulsatile tinnitus is deemed inoperable or present without other concerning clinical findings, tinnitus counseling that emphasizes the benign nature of the pulsing sensation is appropriate.[4]

15.8 Final Diagnosis and Recommended Treatment

WA had a moderate to profound sensorineural hearing loss and pulsatile tinnitus in his left ear. His pulsatile tinnitus only presented itself when wearing his new custom hearing instrument in that ear. After acoustic and physical manipulation of the hearing device, sound therapy was attempted. Sound therapy was not successful with this patient, as the tinnitus was resistant to masking attempts. After a CT angiogram and temporal bone scan were performed, it was found that the patient's left temporal bone between the Eustachian tube and the internal carotid artery was dehiscent, and likely contributing to the sensation of pulsing. The canal portion of the hearing device was tapered as to reduce contact with the ear canal, thereby limiting the device's contribution to the pulsing sensation.

15.9 Outcome

After multiple appointments with the audiologist, and the manufacturer's audiologist, cardiologist, and otolaryngologist, it was found that left temporal bone dehiscence was the root cause of his pulsatile tinnitus when wearing his hearing device. After physical manipulation of the custom hearing instrument, the patient reported satisfaction and relief from his pulsatile tinnitus.

15.10 Clinician Self-Efficacy

- Working with other medical professionals is necessary when a patient is experiencing pulsatile tinnitus to rule out a medically treatable factor or explore further diagnoses.
- Having the ability to physically manipulate a device in office is beneficial for you and the patient.

References

[1] Henry J, Zaugg T, Myers P, Kendall C. Progressive tinnitus management clinical handbook for audiologists. Plural Publishing; 2010

[2] Liyanage SH, Singh A, Savundra P, Kalan A. Pulsatile tinnitus. J Laryngol Otol. 2006; 120(2):93–97

[3] Sismanis A. Pulsatile tinnitus: contemporary assessment and management. Curr Opin Otolaryngol Head Neck Surg. 2011; 19(5):348–357

[4] Rathé M, Govaere F, Forton GEJ. Unilateral pulsatile tinnitus associated with an internal carotid artery-Eustachian tube dehiscence. OTO Open. 2018; 2(1):X17753605

Section A: Medical Cases

II: Disorders of Sound Tolerance

16 Hyperacusis and Military Noise Exposure

LaGuinn P. Sherlock

This is a case report of a 54-year-old active duty service member presenting with complaints of decreased sound tolerance, subjective hearing loss, and constant bilateral tinnitus.

16.1 Clinical History and Description

A 54-year-old patient was seen initially in hearing conservation for a diagnostic audiological evaluation, presenting with a report of sensitivity to sounds such as sirens, vacuum cleaners, and clapping hands. He also reported increased difficulty hearing in the presence of background noise, necessitating frequent requests for repetition. He reported bilateral, constant tinnitus with an initial onset 6 to 8 months prior to the evaluation. He noted that the tinnitus interfered with his ability to get to sleep. History was significant for past military noise exposure (airfields and gunfire).

16.2 Audiological Testing

Standard audiometric testing (see ▶ Fig. 16.1) was conducted by the hearing conservation audiologist. Otoscopic inspection revealed clear ear canals bilaterally. Pure-tone threshold testing indicated a bilateral high-frequency sensorineural hearing loss. Hearing sensitivity was characterized by normal audiometric thresholds from 250 to 3,000 Hz, sloping to a mild hearing loss at 8,000 Hz in both ears. Word recognition scores in quiet were 100% in both ears. Tympanometry revealed normal tympanic membrane/middle ear system compliance and pressure in both ears. Ipsilateral acoustic reflex thresholds were present at normal levels bilaterally. The patient completed the Tinnitus and Hearing Survey (THS).[1] His subscale totals were 5 for tinnitus, 12 for hearing, and 3 for sound tolerance. The patient was subsequently referred for specialty evaluation to address his complaint of reduced sound tolerance.

16.3 Questions for the Reader

1. If a patient reports hypersensitivity to sound, should you measure acoustic reflex thresholds?
2. Based on the patient's THS subscores, which symptom is most problematic?
3. Would you recommend hearing aids at this time?

16.4 Discussion of Questions for the Reader

1. *If a patient reports hypersensitivity to sound, should you measure acoustic reflex thresholds?*
   Patients with reduced sound tolerance may react adversely to the presentation of stimuli at intensity levels sufficient to elicit an acoustic reflex. Caution must be exercised in measuring acoustic reflexes with this population, and if it is determined that reflexes must be tested, then the test should be conducted at the end of the evaluation.
2. *Based on the patient's THS subscores, which symptom is most problematic?*
   The THS is designed to differentiate tinnitus problems, hearing problems, and sound tolerance problems in order to address the primary complaint. The total possible points on the tinnitus and hearing subscales are 16 points each, whereas the total possible score on the sound tolerance subscale is 4. Therefore, the patient's primary concern, according to the THS, is sound tolerance. This is consistent with his subjective report and suggests that sound tolerance issues should be managed prior to the tinnitus and hearing-related complaints.
3. *Would you recommend hearing aids at this time?*
   Patients who present with subjective complaints of hearing loss and bothersome tinnitus and have measurable hearing loss are typically excellent candidates for amplification. However, patients presenting with sound tolerance complaints may require additional evaluation to assess hyperacusis before hearing aids are recommended. The likelihood of a successful hearing aid fitting improves when sound tolerance issues are managed prior to the fitting.

16.5 Final Diagnosis and Recommended Treatment

The patient was seen in the Audiology clinic for a hyperacusis evaluation, during which a detailed

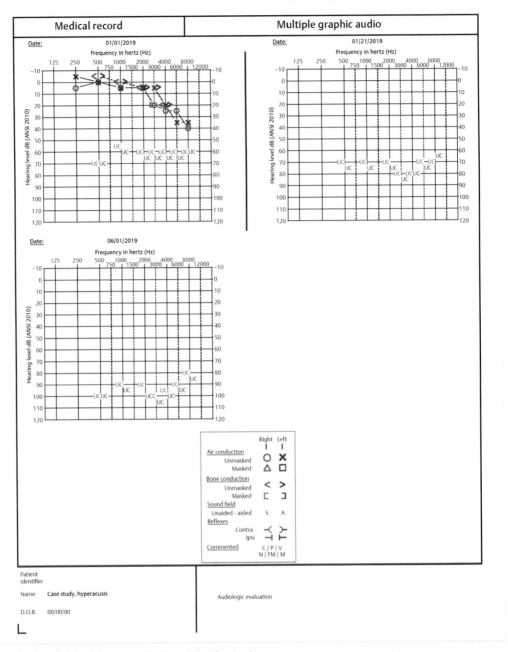

Fig. 16.1 Audiology results. LDLs, loudness discomfort levels.

history regarding his sound sensitivity, tinnitus, and hearing complaints was obtained. The patient reported that while he was deployed in Afghanistan 8 years ago, his quarters were next to an airfield, and the window faced the runway. After being there for a several months, he woke up frequently with pain in his ears. He reported feeling similar pain during exposure to loud sounds over the past year, with a pain rating of 3 to 4 (on a scale of 1–10). Based on the patient's responses during the evaluation, his sound tolerance problems are experienced most frequently at concerts/movie theaters, around children, and while doing housework. The patient reported that loud music, the presence of background noise when trying to listen to someone speak, and the presence of multiple sounds (e.g., people talking, dishes clattering, doors closing, footsteps) bothers him often. The patient described his appropriate use of hearing protection devices during exposure to hazardous sound levels and denied using hearing protection devices to avoid sound in general. The patient described his tinnitus as a high-pitched buzzing sound that primarily affects his ability to hear. His Tinnitus Functional Index score was 33.6, indicating a "significant problem with tinnitus, with a possible/borderline need for professional intervention."[2]

Subjectively, the patient rated the severity of his sound tolerance problem at 7 (0 = not a problem; 10 = as big a problem as one can imagine). He rated the effect of reduced sound tolerance on his life at 3 (0 = no effect; 10 = as big an effect as one can imagine) and the distress caused by reduced sound tolerance at 3 (0 = no distress; 10 = as much distress as one can imagine). Loudness discomfort levels (LDLs) were measured for pure tones and ranged from 55 to 65 dB HL in the frequency region of 500 to 8,000 Hz, in both ears. Based on the pattern of LDLs (high-frequency LDLs converging with audiometric thresholds, rather than LDLs paralleling audiometric thresholds)[3] and the patient's subjective report of sensitivity to the loudness of sound rather than sensitivity to particular sounds, he was judged to have clinically significant hyperacusis. Ear-level sound therapy was recommended to the patient, and he agreed with the recommendation.

Sound therapy was implemented using open-fit, receiver-in-the-canal hearing aids with masking circuitry. Probe microphone measurements were conducted to verify appropriate sound generator output. When the hearing aids were programmed to emit broadband noise (500–4,000 Hz) and the volume was set to 44 dBSPL in the programming software, the patient judged the volume to be "comfortable but soft." At this level, the device output did not exceed the noise floor of the room. The volume was subsequently adjusted to 49 dBSPL and the frequency range of the noise was adjusted to 500 to 4,000 Hz. The patient verified the sound was not annoying and the devices were comfortable. The patient was instructed to use the sound generators every day for a minimum of 8 hours per day.

16.6 Additional Questions for the Reader

1. Why is it important to determine whether patients with sound tolerance complaints are overprotecting their hearing?
2. Is there evidence that LDLs can be measured reliably?
3. Why is it important to verify the patient-selected volume of the sound generators?

16.7 Discussion of Additional Questions for the Reader

1. *Why is it important to determine whether patients with sound tolerance complaints are overprotecting their hearing?*
   Frequent use of hearing protection devices to avoid sound can exacerbate sound sensitivity. Changes in LDLs have been observed in research participants without sound sensitivity as a function of external sound. When earplugs were used continuously over a period of 1 to 2 weeks, LDLs were lower than baseline. Conversely, when sound generators were used continuously for weeks, LDLs were higher than baseline.[4,5] Elevations in LDLs have been observed clinically in patients undergoing sound therapy.[6]
2. *Is there evidence that LDLs can be measured reliably?*
   It is generally believed that different methodologies for obtaining LDLs can result in significantly different estimates. However, there is evidence that LDL estimates are comparable using relative and absolute measurements of loudness.[7] As long as the clinical method is consistent, LDLs can be measured with good reliability. Treatment progress can be evaluated using a combination of LDLs and subjective reports.
3. *Why is it important to verify the patient-selected volume of the sound generators?*
   If the volume is set too low, then sound therapy is unlikely to be beneficial. When patients describe the sound generator volume as "soft" or "comfortable but soft," it may be insufficient to have a treatment effect. Therefore, it is important to verify that the sound generator volume is above the noise floor of the room. With open fittings, the target is at least 5 to 7 dB of insertion gain in the frequency region of

2 to 4 kHz. Based on clinical observation, and for the goal of improving loudness tolerance, this level is sufficient. In addition, probe microphone measurements are helpful as a counseling tool to demonstrate the reason for volume adjustments (i.e., to a level above the noise floor). When setting the sound generator parameters, it is important to ensure the sound is tolerable. Most hyperacusic patients prefer less high-frequency energy (e.g., pink noise rather than white noise).

16.8 Outcome

The patient returned to the clinic 3 weeks after sound therapy was initiated, and he reported daily use of the sound generators. LDLs were remeasured and shifted to 65 to 85 dB HL. Subjectively, the patient noticed an improvement in his ability to tolerate sounds. Five months later, his sound tolerance levels shifted further to 85 to 105 dB HL, his sound tolerance severity rating decreased to 3, and his THS sound tolerance subscore decreased to 1. The hearing aid microphones were activated to address his complaint of subjective hearing loss. Three months later, he reported situational use of amplification and continued use of sound therapy. His THS scores were 5/16 for tinnitus, 0/16 for hearing, and 0.5/4 for sound tolerance.

16.9 Self-Efficacy for Clinicians

It is easy to question the legitimacy of LDLs that are 55 to 65 dB HL when the patient appears to be able to tolerate normal conversational levels. Keep in mind: many people with hyperacusis also have some degree of phonophobia, which may result in LDLs that are lower than what the patient can actually tolerate. That is why it is important to spend time talking to the patient to find out how the reduced sound tolerance is affecting them in daily life. When there are reports of activity limitations and reduced LDLs, sound therapy can be very helpful. The goal with sound therapy is to provide a low-volume level of continuous sound. There has been no systematic study of the "correct" volume to set the sound generators. The recommendation for 5 to 7 dB above the noise floor is based on clinical protocol and a high rate of success in getting patients back to normal everyday functioning. Sometimes clinicians want to jump in with hearing

aids because of hearing loss and subjective hearing difficulty, but in a patient with low LDLs, the likelihood of hearing aid rejection is high. Spending a few months with sound therapy alone can facilitate hearing aid success (see Suggested Readings).

Acknowledgment

The author would like to thank Sienna Software Inc. for providing the AudBase audiogram form.

References

[1] Henry JA, Griest S, Zaugg TL, et al. Tinnitus and hearing survey: a screening tool to differentiate bothersome tinnitus from hearing difficulties. Am J Audiol. 2015; 24(1):66–77

[2] Meikle MB, Henry JA, Griest SE, et al. The tinnitus functional index: development of a new clinical measure for chronic, intrusive tinnitus. Ear Hear. 2012; 33(2):153–176

[3] Jastreboff PJ, Jastreboff MM. Tinnitus retraining therapy for management of tinnitus and hyperacusis. Seminar presented in Columbia, MD; 2010

[4] Formby C, Sherlock LP, Gold SL. Adaptive plasticity of loudness induced by chronic attenuation and enhancement of the acoustic background. J Acoust Soc Am. 2003; 114(1):55–58

[5] Formby C, Sherlock LP, Gold SL, Hawley ML. Adaptive recalibration of chronic auditory gain. Semin Hear. 2007; 28:295–302

[6] Formby C, Gold SL. Modification of loudness discomfort level: evidence for adaptive chronic auditory gain and its clinical relevance. Semin Hear. 2002; 23:21–34

[7] Sherlock LP, Formby C. Estimates of loudness, loudness discomfort, and the auditory dynamic range: normative estimates, comparison of procedures, and test-retest reliability. J Am Acad Audiol. 2005; 16(2):85–100

Suggested Readings

Formby C, Hawley ML, Sherlock LP, et al. A sound therapy-based intervention to expand the auditory dynamic range for loudness among persons with sensorineural hearing losses: a randomized placebo-controlled clinical trial. Semin Hear. 2015; 36(2):77–110

Formby C, Sherlock LP, Hawley ML, Gold SL, Gold S. A sound therapy-based intervention to expand the auditory dynamic range for loudness among persons with sensorineural hearing losses: case evidence showcasing treatment efficacy. Semin Hear. 2017; 38(1):130–150

Disclaimer

The view expressed is that of the author and does not reflect the official policy of the U.S. Departments of the Army, Navy, and Air Force; the U.S. Department of Defense; or the U.S. Government.

17 Diplacusis or the Affected Audiologist

Marc Fagelson

17.1 Background

The patient, a 57-year-old male audiologist, sought clinical services for a sudden sensorineural hearing loss (SSNHL) in the right ear, noticed upon waking, on March 15, 2016. Audiometric history included decades of recreational exposure to recorded and amplified music, no substantial occupational noise, and no military service. The ear reportedly felt "full" the night before; however, the patient reported that such a sensation was not unprecedented, and that he did not expect to awake with an obvious, unilateral, change in threshold. Also apparent upon waking was bilateral white noise tinnitus lateralized somewhat to the right. Patient reported experiencing intermittent tinnitus for more than 40 years, usually immediately following exposures to amplified music and/or noisy environments. In the past, tinnitus reportedly appeared in response to environmental sounds or spontaneously for bursts of 1 to 2 minutes (i.e., sudden brief unilateral tapering tinnitus [SBUTT][1]). At the time of the appointment, the patient reported constant tinnitus in addition to a "cellophane" crackling sensation when sound was directed to the affected ear. No vestibular symptoms nor sound tolerance issues were reported.

17.2 Assessment

The patient measured an audiogram early the same morning the hearing loss appeared. Pure-tone air conduction testing revealed normal thresholds in the left ear and a severe sensorineural hearing loss sloping from 1 to 8 kHz in the right ear (▶ Table 17.1). Weber lateralized to the left at 1 and 2 kHz. Bone conduction and immittance testing were not conducted. The loss was consistent with a sensorineural site of lesion, as in addition

to the Weber result, the patient determined that phonation of the vowel /a/ increased in loudness when he occluded either ear, a finding similar to that of a positive (no conductive component) Bing test.

The patient was seen later in the day for a brief otolaryngological workup. He shared the audiometric results obtained hours earlier and after consultation, was prescribed prednisone, and returned to work. Sounds remained muffled and "crackly" in the right ear, although no word recognition testing was conducted. The patient also noticed that environmental sounds produced a similar crackling sensation as that produced by speech. After returning home, the patient listened to music while alternately plugging the good ear and the affected ear. In all cases, the music appeared to shift upward in pitch by a full step when the patient plugged the good ear. When plugging the affected ear, the music sounded natural and retained its original pitch.

17.3 Questions for the Reader

1. What are the essential questions to ask the patient who reports a sudden hearing loss?
2. How soon after noticing a sudden hearing loss will intervention have the potential to provide a positive outcome?
3. How does diplacusis present?

17.4 Answers to Questions for the Reader

1. *What are the essential questions to ask the patient who reports a sudden hearing loss?*
   Patients who experience sudden hearing loss may report tinnitus, vestibular problems, and

Table 17.1 Pure-tone thresholds (dB HL) before (pre-PT) and after (3/15/16) sudden hearing loss onset. AD: right ear; AS: left ear

	250 Hz	500 Hz	1000 Hz	1500 Hz	2000 Hz	3000 Hz	4000 Hz	6000 Hz	8000 Hz
Pre-PT AD	10	20	15		20	25	30	30	35
AD: 3/15/16	20	25	30	35	45	55	75	80	80
Current	20	15	20	20	30	30	45	45	40
Pre-PT AS	15	10	15		15	10	15	15	20
AS: 3/15/16/	15	20	15		15	20	25	20	25

difficulty communicating in familiar settings. The progression of the loss is important to determine its laterality, and its effects should all be discussed. The severity of tinnitus can be determined using a validated intake instrument, such as the Tinnitus Functional Index (TFI)[2] or the Tinnitus Handicap Inventory (THI).[3] Patients may note that sounds and voices no longer sound natural, and it is reasonable to provide the opportunity for patients to report such changes. Some patients will be aware that specific sounds, such as music, no longer maintain their familiar pitch or timbre, and a conversation re: music listening and expectations may support the patient continuing to listen as a way to manage the pitch anomalies associated with diplacusis.

2. *How soon after noticing a sudden hearing loss will intervention have the potential to provide a positive outcome?*
   According to the AAO-HNS guidelines,[4] early intervention is most likely to produce a positive outcome. The guideline indicates that audiometric confirmation of SSNHL should take place within 14 days of the observed change in hearing. In addition, the use of corticosteroids, if indicated, should occur within 14 days of the SSNHL onset. Therefore, after ruling out a conductive component to the sudden loss, the patient has approximately 14 days from the onset of the loss to seek the standard steroid treatment as prescribed by an ENT physician.

3. *How does diplacusis present?*
   The most typical presentation of diplacusis in the literature features the sensation of one sound (i.e., a pure-tone or musical passage), producing a different pitch sensation across the two ears. For example, a pure tone of 1,000 Hz might evoke the 1,000-Hz pitch in one ear while producing the sensation of an 1,100-Hz tone in the other ear. A song in the key of C might generate the perception of being the key of D (or a full step higher in pitch) in an affected ear. Some patients can map out frequency regions in which pitch sensations are as expected even as they depart from the expected pitch in other regions.

17.5 Outcome

Within 48 hours after starting prednisone, the patient observed that sound in the affected ear returned to its pre-event clarity, although the sensitivity in the ear remained outside the normal range. The patient continued working, socializing, and listening to music through the time period during which the hearing partially returned, and the diplacusis sensation faded within the same 48-hour time period.

17.6 Clinician Self-Efficacy

The paucity of diplacusis cases suggests that interventions and symptom management will be difficult to study systematically. In some cases, the affected individual is a musician; the patient may bring to the clinic a map, perhaps a drawing of a piano keyboard, to illustrate the notes for which their pitch experience is not normal. In the past 20 years, the author worked with two patients who presented with diplacusis, both were musicians, and both had to some degree given up writing, performing, and listening to music. The patients were encouraged to find and consume musical passages in keys that were least affected by the diplacusis. Neither patient experienced complete remission of the diplacusis sensation at 6 months postcounseling, and both struggled at times with the symptom. Other patients with diplacusis experienced different outcomes, in particular, one patient reported upon by Reiss et al.[5] As a result of Reiss's work, it is reasonable to ask:

17.6.1 Can Sound Enrichment Facilitate Recovery from Diplacusis?

Although the value of desensitization for reduced loudness tolerance and dynamic range is well established,[6] the same cannot be said with certainty regarding diplacusis. Reiss et al[5] demonstrated substantial changes in pitch perception in patients who received cochlear implants. She reported a patient who received a hybrid implant in one ear, then years later, a full-length electrode array in the other ear. After receiving the second implant, the patient lost all hearing in the ear originally fitted with a short-electrode hybrid. Pitch perception at each ear differed substantially for years; however, during that time the patient maintained consistent use of both implants. After approximately 3 years of such use, the patient's pitch perception to a 1,000-Hz tone returned binaurally despite the presence of a sudden onset profound deafness in the ear that was fitted years earlier with the hybrid, short-electrode device. The patient could pitch match a 1,000-Hz tone in each ear despite lacking an electrode at the 1,000-Hz place in the cochlea in the right ear.

Perhaps the rule of thumb here is that if the patient changes nothing, then the patient should expect their condition to remain unchanged. If the patient has hearing loss, then an assistive device or hearing aid offers a reasonable starting point. Stimulating the pathway by enriching the presence of external sound may be a challenge for patients whose sound world and relationship with music and conversation is altered. For some patients, a diplacusis symptom poses an occupational, if not existential threat. Collaborating with the patient to find sound/music that is least objectionable may provide an avenue toward understanding the patient's situation, as well as supporting the patient's acceptance that the symptom, although real, may be amenable to modification through various listening strategies.

References

[1] Oron Y, Roth Y, Levine RA. Sudden brief unilateral tapering tinnitus: prevalence and properties. Otol Neurotol. 2011; 32 (9):1409–1414

[2] Meikle MB, Henry JA, Griest SE, et al. The tinnitus functional index: development of a new clinical measure for chronic, intrusive tinnitus. Ear Hear. 2012; 33(2):153–176

[3] Newman CW, Jacobson GP, Spitzer JB. Development of the tinnitus handicap inventory. Arch Otolaryngol Head Neck Surg. 1996; 122(2):143–148

[4] Chandrasekhar SS, Tsai Do BS, Schwartz SR, et al. Clinical practice guideline: sudden hearing loss (update). Otolaryngol Head Neck Surg. 2019; 161(1):1–45– American Academy of Otolaryngology–Head and Neck Surgery Foundation

[5] Reiss LAJ, Lowder MW, Karsten SA, Turner CW, Gantz BJ. Effects of extreme tonotopic mismatches between bilateral cochlear implants on electric pitch perception: a case study. Ear Hear. 2011; 32(4):536–540

[6] Formby C, Sherlock LP, Gold SL. Adaptive plasticity of loudness induced by chronic attenuation and enhancement of the acoustic background. J Acoust Soc Am. 2003; 114(1): 55–58

Section B: Psychological Correlates

I: Tinnitus

18 Tinnitus and Misophonia in an Adolescent Patient

Suzanne H. Kimball

18.1 Clinical History and Description

PE, an 18-year-old female, was referred to our university tinnitus clinic by a local pediatric otolaryngologist for evaluation of her tinnitus and sound sensitivity symptoms. The patient reported that her tinnitus began when she was 8 years old. She indicated that her tinnitus became painfully loud when she was in a quiet environment. In addition, PE reported significant sound sensitivity to specific sounds like chewing, heavy breathing, or yawning, particularly when these sounds were produced by her parents. It was reported that the patient was known to isolate herself at home due to irritation from these sounds. PE's mother was present in the room for the initial interview and all testing procedures. Both PE and her mother cried when she described her sound sensitivity. Both concluded that the sensitivity had a significant negative impact on her quality of life and their overall family dynamic.

18.2 Audiological Testing

PE received a comprehensive audiological evaluation at the referring doctor's office approximately 3 weeks prior to her appointment in the university clinic. Pure-tone test results from the prior evaluation indicated normal hearing sensitivity for both ears from 250 to 8,000 Hz. Speech recognition thresholds were established at 15 dB HL for both ears with 100% word recognition scores. Twelve-frequency distortion product otoacoustic emissions (DPOAEs) were present in both ears. Tympanometry indicated bilateral normal, type A tympanograms. Ipsilateral acoustic reflexes were present in the right ear but were absent in the left ear (▶ Fig. 18.1).

18.3 Questions for the Reader

1. What additional case history information might be pertinent to this case?
2. What additional audiological testing would be recommended?
3. What is misophonia?

4. Why is it that hearing certain sounds can produce such powerful physical reactions?
5. What treatment options might be considered?

18.4 Discussion of Questions for the Reader

1. *What additional case history information might be pertinent to this case?*
   It would be important to determine the severity of the tinnitus complaint, when the condition began to worsen, and whether the patient could identify any event associated with the tinnitus exacerbation. It would also be helpful to determine whether there were any coexisting medical or psychological conditions (such as anxiety and/or depression), the specific life activities (i.e., sleep, concentration) affected by tinnitus, and how the current tinnitus and misophonia symptoms were being managed (if at all).

2. *What additional audiological testing would be recommended?*
   Additional audiological measures could include the following:
   a) High-frequency pure-tone thresholds measured bilaterally from 9,000 to 20,000 Hz to identify hearing loss outside of the standard testing frequencies.
   b) A complete tinnitus evaluation for each affected ear(s) including pitch match, loudness match, minimum masking level for white and/or narrow band noise, and residual inhibition is optional; however, it can be carried out at the family's request. Of these measures, minimum masking level would be most informative, as it would provide evidence that the tinnitus could be masked by external sound.
   c) Loudness discomfort levels (LDLs) measured for each ear using pure tones (500, 1,000, 2,000, and 4,000 Hz) and speech (monitored live voice) stimuli. This is to determine loudness tolerance for both speech and pure-tone stimulation.
   d) Validated scales of tinnitus including the Tinnitus Handicap Inventory (THI)[1] and the

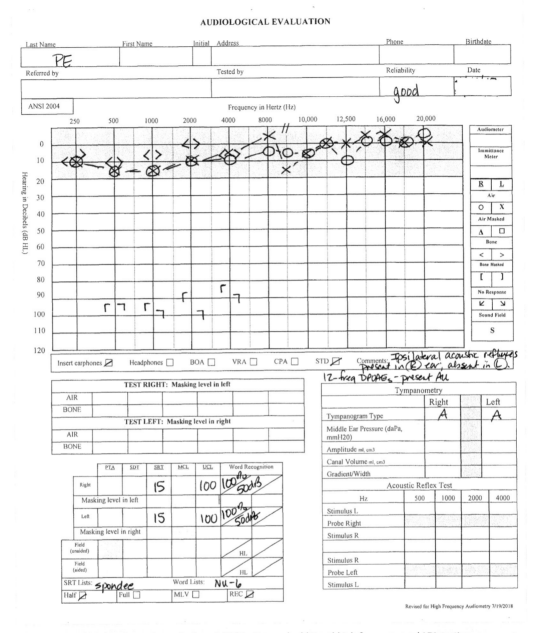

Fig. 18.1 Combined audiometric results from initial testing and additional high-frequency and LDL testing.

Tinnitus Functional Index (TFI)[2] to monitor severity and the impact on quality of life; and subjective scales of misophonia such as the Amsterdam Misophonia Scale (A-MISO)[3] to assess the patient's aversion to specific sounds.

3. *What is misophonia?*

The term "misophonia" translates as "hatred of sound"[4] and is characterized as a chronic condition in which specific sounds provoke intense emotional experiences and autonomic arousal within the individual.[5] Misophonia, or annoyance hyperacusis in Tyler et al's[6] classification scheme, may be present along with tinnitus.[7] Jastreboff and Hazell[8] propose that misophonia and tinnitus are both associated with hyperconnectivity between the auditory and limbic systems.[5] With misophonia, or annoyance hyperacusis, the physical characteristics of a sound are secondary, with the more significant element being the patient's previous history with the sounds' sources, or the sounds themselves.[7] The most common sound triggers are known to be those produced by humans such as chewing, breathing, and lip smacking. In some cases, visual triggers may be present; for example, a video of a person chewing or the repeated tapping of a pen or the pressing of a pen or pencil to expose the tip may amplify or provoke the negative response. Individuals with misophonia may become so disturbed by the presence of the triggering sounds that they may isolate themselves from social situations. Individuals with annoyance hyperacusis most commonly report anxiety, panic, and rage when exposed to triggering sounds.[5]

4. *Why is it that hearing certain sounds can produce such powerful physical reactions?*
Kumar et al[9] demonstrated brain activity in misophonic patients commensurate with powerful fight or flight responses to trigger sounds that was not observed in unaffected individuals. Kumar showed that trigger sounds produced significantly more activity in auditory and emotional centers of misophonic individual's brains than age and hearing-matched nonmisophonic controls, while neutral sounds, such as rain falling, produced similar responses across the two groups. This finding may help to explain why individuals with misophonia show strong emotional and physical reactions, such as anger and avoidance, when confronted by the triggers.

5. *What treatment options might be considered?*
Based on the Jastreboff protocol for Tinnitus Retraining Therapy (TRT), or Cima and colleagues[10] use of cognitive behavioral therapy (CBT), tinnitus can be managed with a systematic program of sound therapy and counseling. In TRT, sound therapy is delivered across a range of signal levels below the so-called "mixing point," which is defined as the level at which a masking sound partially masks the audible tinnitus. Jastreboff and Jastreboff[7] also developed a systematic program for the management of misophonia including a four-level process geared toward creating a positive association with a sound and the use of sound generators to interfere with, but not cover up the offending sounds.

18.5 Additional Testing

High-frequency audiometry was completed bilaterally from 9,000 to 20,000 Hz. The results of this testing indicated hearing thresholds better than 15 dB HL for all test frequencies for both ears.

LDLs were obtained separately for each ear at the pure-tone frequencies of 500, 1,000, 2,000, and 4,000 Hz as well as for monitored live voice. LDLs were consistently established between 85 and 100 dB HL, which was considered evidence of slightly reduced sound tolerance at only 2,000 and 4,000 Hz. Her speech LDL was established at 100 dB HL for both ears. Sherlock and Formby[11] indicated that LDLs for adults with normal hearing should be 95 dB HL or higher (▶ Fig. 18.1).

During the intake interview, PE subjectively scored the severity of her tinnitus as 9 out of 10, annoyance as a 9/10, and the overall effect on her quality of life as a 7/10.

The patient scored a 54/100 on the THI and a 60/100 on the TFI, indicating that she was moderately bothered by her tinnitus symptoms. In particular, the patient rated as most severe her inability to concentrate and to focus attention. She indicated that she was aware of tinnitus about 70 to 80% of the time and was annoyed by it 100% of the time when she was aware of it. The A-MISO was not available during this appointment and therefore was not administered. Misophonia triggers were discussed with her during the initial intake interview. As indicated, her primary misophonia triggers were chewing, smacking, heavy breathing, and yawning, particularly when these sounds were produced by her parents.

18.6 Additional Questions for the Reader

1. What other medical factors should be taken into account for this patient?
2. What other measurements or considerations might be included to determine the patient's level of anxiety, depression, or other mental health factors?

18.7 Discussion of Additional Questions for the Reader

1. *What other medical factors should be taken into account for this patient?*
Even with PE's young age, she presented with a

significant medical history, including removal of a thyroid mass, subsequently diagnosed in pathology reports as Hashimoto thyroiditis. Hashimoto thyroiditis is an autoimmune disease in which the immune system attacks the thyroid gland. Clinical findings include enlargement of the thyroid gland, fatigue, weight gain, sensitivity to cold, joint and muscle pain, abnormal menstrual periods, depression, and slowed heart rate.[12] Of note for audiological consideration is the presence of an autoimmune disorder, which can affect the inner ear, and the increased likelihood of depression, which can exacerbate sound sensitivity and tinnitus symptoms.

2. *What other measurements or considerations might be included to determine the patient's level of anxiety, depression, or other mental health factors?* The Beck Depression Inventory (BDI)[13] and the Hospital Anxiety and Depression Scale (HADS)[14] are two examples of questionnaires that could be administered as screening measurements for anxiety and depression. Based on the scores, a mental health referral could be indicated. PE did appear concerned about her tinnitus and sound sensitivity, particularly evident in her desire to withdraw from social situations. She regularly attended a public high school, reportedly had ample friends, and routinely attended social activities typical for her age group. Brout et al[15] emphasized the value of interprofessional care: "providers should adopt a multi-disciplinary approach to the assessment and intervention of misophonia and co-occurring physical and behavioral health problems" (p. 10).

18.8 Final Diagnosis and Recommended Treatment

Clinic protocol suggested the use of TRT in order to address co-occurrence of symptoms associated with both annoyance hyperacusis and tinnitus. TRT is a form of habituation therapy designed by Jastreboff and Hazell[8] to reduce the effects of tinnitus on affected individuals. Two key components of TRT directly follow from the neurophysiological model of tinnitus.[16] One of these principles includes directive counseling that prioritizes the patient's reclassification of tinnitus from a sound that evokes concern to one that is neutral, while the other element of management includes sound therapy intended to weaken tinnitus-related neuronal activity. Because there was no evidence of hearing loss for this patient and insurance would not cover the cost of hearing devices, it was recommended

that the sound therapy be delivered via an application (app) on her smartphone.

18.9 Additional Questions for the Reader

1. Is tinnitus management best supported through tinnitus maskers or combination hearing aid devices?
2. What follow-up testing is recommended?

18.10 Discussion of Additional Questions for the Reader

1. *Is tinnitus management best supported through tinnitus maskers or combination hearing aid devices?*
   The short answer to this question is, "both is best." Traditional tinnitus maskers are ear-level devices that provide constant stimulation of broadband noise whose volume can be controlled by the user. These devices do not provide amplification. Combination devices, on the other hand, have the advantage of providing amplification when needed but can also have tinnitus masking noise (sound therapy) added to a program with amplification, as a standalone program, or streamed to aids if the devices are smartphone compatible. Obviously, the advantage of a combination device is its provision of prescribed amplification to the listener as well as masking sound for tinnitus relief. When a patient is not a good candidate for a hearing aid, a tinnitus masker may provide adequate tinnitus relief and can often be purchased at a lower price. With the emergence of smartphone technology however, dozens of tinnitus applications, "apps," are now available, often free, and include relaxing and therapeutic sounds that may be comparable with tinnitus masking devices. Patients can stream sounds from the app through their personal earphones or earbuds. Hesse[17] and Sereda et al[18] suggest that apps can be a useful supplement to the myriad of available tinnitus therapies.
2. *What follow-up testing is recommended?*
   Patients should be followed approximately every 3 months for up to 18 months to determine (1) whether tinnitus habituation was achieved and (2) if the sound sensitivity decreased. Audiometric measures should be repeated at the 6-month appointment.

18.11 Self-Advocacy Tips

- Patients may present to a clinic with a variety of symptoms including tinnitus, hyperacusis, and misophonia.
- Treatment options for all of these conditions are viable.
- A team approach for the treatment of misophonia is optimal, including audiology, neurology, and psychology.

References

[1] Newman CW, Jacobson GP, Spitzer JB. Development of the Tinnitus Handicap Inventory. Arch Otolaryngol Head Neck Surg. 1996; 122(2):143–148

[2] Meikle MB, Henry JA, Griest SE, et al. The tinnitus functional index: development of a new clinical measure for chronic, intrusive tinnitus. Ear Hear. 2012; 33(2):153–176

[3] Schröder A, Vulink N, Denys D. Misophonia: diagnostic criteria for a new psychiatric disorder. PLoS One. 2013; 8(1):e54706

[4] Jastreboff MM, Jastreboff PJ. Components of decreased sound tolerance: hyperacusis, misophonia, phonophobia. ITHS News Lett.. 2001; 2:5–7

[5] Edelstein M, Brang D, Rouw R, Ramachandran VS. Misophonia: physiological investigations and case descriptions. Front Hum Neurosci. 2013; 7:296

[6] Tyler RS, Pienkowski M, Roncancio ER, et al. A review of hyperacusis and future directions: part I. Definitions and manifestations. Am J Audiol. 2014; 23(4):402–419

[7] Jastreboff MM, Jastreboff PJ. Decreased sound tolerance and tinnitus retraining therapy (TRT). Aust N Z J Audiol. 2002; 24: 74–84

[8] Jastreboff PJ, Hazell J. Tinnitus retraining therapy: implementing the neurophysiological model. Cambridge University Press; 2004

[9] Kumar S, Tansley-Hancock O, Sedley W, et al. The brain basis for misophonia. Curr Biol. 2017; 27(4):527–533

[10] Cima RF, Maes IH, Joore MA, et al. Specialised treatment based on cognitive behaviour therapy versus usual care for tinnitus: a randomised controlled trial. Lancet. 2012; 379 (9830):1951–1959

[11] Sherlock LP, Formby C. Estimates of loudness, loudness discomfort, and the auditory dynamic range: normative estimates, comparison of procedures, and test-retest reliability. J Am Acad Audiol. 2005; 16(2):85–100

[12] Web MD. Hashimoto's Thyroiditis Directory; 2018. Retrieved July 18, 2018 from https://www.webmd.com/women/hashimotos-thyroiditis-directory

[13] Beck AT, Ward CH, Mendelson M, Mock J, Erbaugh J. An inventory for measuring depression. Arch Gen Psychiatry. 1961; 4:561–571

[14] Zigmond AS, Snaith RP. The hospital anxiety and depression scale. Acta Psychiatr Scand. 1983; 67(6):361–370

[15] Brout JJ, Edelstein M, Erfanian M, et al. Investigating misophonia: a review of the empirical literature, clinical implications, and a research agenda. Front Neurosci. 2018; 12:36

[16] Jastreboff PJ. Phantom auditory perception (tinnitus): mechanisms of generation and perception. Neurosci Res. 1990; 8(4):221–254

[17] Hesse G. Smartphone app-supported approaches to tinnitus therapy. HNO. 2018; 66(5):350–357

[18] Sereda M, Smith S, Newton K, Stockdale D. Mobile apps for management of tinnitus: users' survey, quality assessment, and content analysis. JMIR Mhealth Uhealth. 2019; 7(1): e10353

19 Severe Hyperacusis and Tinnitus

Erin Benear and Isabella Hillerby

19.1 Clinical History and Description

BJ is a 56-year-old female seen at a University Speech and Hearing Center with the chief complaint of severe sound intolerance and bilateral tinnitus. Case history indicated high-frequency hearing loss identified at an ENT appointment 2 months prior to this date's contact. The Physician's Assistant (PA) diagnosed BJ with hyperacusis and referred her to our clinic. When she arrived at the clinic, BJ chose to wait in the restroom for her appointment because the "sounds in the waiting room were incredibly bothersome." In the test suite, BJ flinched at environmental sounds, including the door opening/closing, placement of the otoscope on the counter, and hearing clinician voices at a normal speaking volume.

She stated her sound intolerance began approximately 1 year ago and worsened substantially with the abrupt onset of her tinnitus 2 months before this appointment. Although the onset of her tinnitus and worsening of hyperacusis occurred during the COVID-19 mandated quarantine, upon question of co-occurring life events, BJ denied the quarantine to have played any role in the development of tinnitus and exacerbation of hyperacusis. BJ reported that despite using a phone app sound generator, sound intolerance and tinnitus reduced her ability to sleep through the night and negatively affected her ability to concentrate on daily tasks. Because "eating sounds cause the tinnitus to become unbearable," she has been unable to chew/swallow most foods, resulting in significant weight-loss. However, BJ reported tinnitus to not be her primary concern at this appointment.

BJ's initial interview indicated sound intolerance exerted a catastrophic (10/10) effect on her life. BJ revealed she removed all sources of sound from her home, wore ear protection some of the time in quiet, and was fearful in anticipation of loud sounds. Upon asking for a reference point for loud sounds, BJ described any sound about the level of a car passing by and louder to be too loud. She also stated her tinnitus becomes reactive when exposed to loud sounds, when eating, and when touching her face/hair/ears. Further, her description of triggering sounds and activities, paired with her subjective report of sleeping problems are consistent with the Diagnostic and Statistical Manual of Mental Disorders Fifth Edition (DSM 5) criteria for anxiety disorder.[1]

19.2 Audiological Testing

BJ was initially seen at an otolaryngology practice for an audiological evaluation. Results indicated a mild-to-moderate hearing loss at 8,000 Hz, bilaterally (▶ Fig. 19.1). At the time of that evaluation, the PA diagnosed her with hyperacusis and referred her to our speech and hearing clinic. BJ reported not understanding her diagnosis of hyperacusis at the time of that appointment and she subsequently researched the condition on her own. Her hearing evaluation just 2 months prior to this visit obviated the need for a complete audiological evaluation. Otoscopy was unremarkable. Due to reported sound intolerance and reactive tinnitus, acoustic immittance testing was not completed.

19.3 Tinnitus Evaluation

In addition to our clinic's tinnitus case history paperwork, BJ completed the Tinnitus Functional Index (TFI)[2] and the Tinnitus Handicap Inventory (THI).[3] BJ scored an 83 on the TFI (very big problem) and an 84 on the THI (catastrophic handicap). Ultra-high-frequency audiometry revealed a moderate-to-severe loss from 9,000 to 14,000 Hz, with no responses above 14,000 Hz. Loudness discomfort levels (LDL) were completed and indicated significantly reduced tolerance bilaterally (45–55 dB HL for speech and 20–30 dB HL 500–4,000 Hz for pure tones; ▶ Fig. 19.2). A tinnitus evaluation was completed, including pitch and loudness match, minimum masking for narrowband and wideband noise, and residual inhibition. Residual inhibition was stopped at 24 seconds due to patient discomfort, but BJ reported some relief following test cessation.

19.4 Questions for the Reader

1. Do you think acoustic immittance testing could have provided useful objective information in this case?

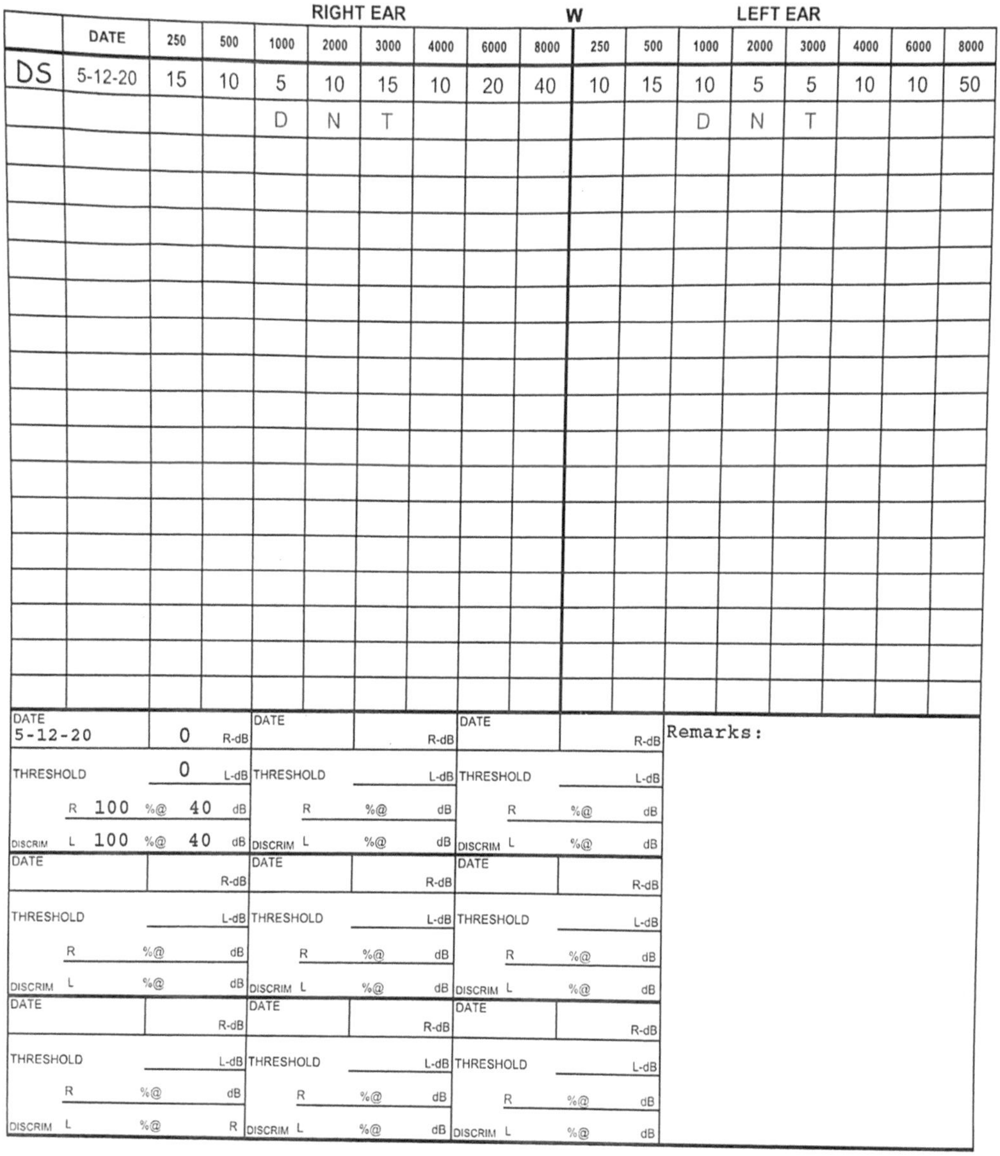

	DATE	250	500	1000	2000	3000	4000	6000	8000	250	500	1000	2000	3000	4000	6000	8000
					RIGHT EAR					**W**				**LEFT EAR**			
DS	5-12-20	15	10	5	10	15	10	20	40	10	15	10	5	5	10	10	50
				D	N	T						D	N	T			

DATE 5-12-20	0	R-dB	DATE		R-dB	DATE		R-dB	Remarks:
THRESHOLD	0	L-dB	THRESHOLD		L-dB	THRESHOLD		L-dB	
	R 100 %@ 40 dB		R %@ dB			R %@ dB			
DISCRIM L 100 %@ 40 dB			DISCRIM L %@ dB			DISCRIM L %@ dB			
DATE		R-dB	DATE		R-dB	DATE		R-dB	
THRESHOLD		L-dB	THRESHOLD		L-dB	THRESHOLD		L-dB	
	R %@ dB		R %@ dB			R %@ dB			
DISCRIM L %@ dB			DISCRIM L %@ dB			DISCRIM L %@ dB			
DATE		R-dB	DATE		R-dB	DATE		R-dB	
THRESHOLD		L-dB	THRESHOLD		L-dB	THRESHOLD		L-dB	
	R %@ dB		R %@ dB			R %@ dB			
DISCRIM L %@ R			DISCRIM L %@ dB			DISCRIM L %@ dB			

Fig. 19.1 Audiogram from previous appointment at an ENT office.

2. How should LDLs be interpreted for this patient?
3. What other case history information would be useful?
4. What management options would you recommend?
5. What medical professional(s) would you recommend her to see?

19.5 Discussion of Questions for the Reader

1. *Do you think acoustic immittance testing could have provided useful objective information in this case?*

It is unlikely that acoustic immittance testing would have provided additional useful

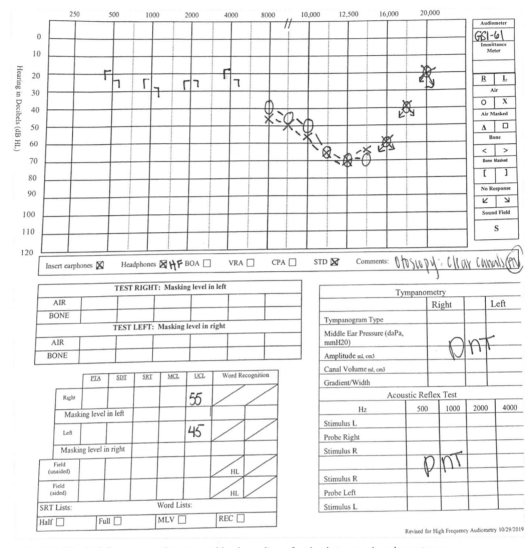

Fig. 19.2 Ultra-high-frequency audiometry and loudness discomfort levels to speech and pure tones.

information in the case of this patient. Completion of immittance testing may have introduced offending sounds/sensations to the patient which could reduce established rapport between the patient and clinicians. Acoustic immittance testing may have exacerbated BJ's tinnitus, as her tinnitus was indicated to be reactive during case history.

2. *How should LDLs be interpreted for this patient?* LDLs are difficult to interpret for patients with and without hyperacusis, particularly LDLs to tones. BJ's LDL response to speech stimuli was recorded at 45 and 55 dB HL; however, her LDLs to tones were significantly lower. Because we do

not live in a world of tones, tonal signals may be perceived as louder than speech, resulting in lower LDLs than we may expect. However, BJ's tolerance seemed to get worse as the appointment progressed. It is possible BJ began lowering her response levels to avoid potentially offensive intensity levels, as she reported a fear of loud sounds at the start of the appointment. In cases such as this, patients may anticipate the next presentation of a sound to be uncomfortably loud, and therefore indicate the current softer presentation level to be at their LDL.[4] Careful instructions and reassuring the patient that all care will be taken to ensure signal levels do not exceed true levels of discomfort may result in more accurate and replicable LDL responses.

3. *What other case history information would be useful?*

   Based on BJ's reported sensations related to her hyperacusis and tinnitus, a history of psychological symptoms or treatments may have been useful. It also would be interesting to have a discussion based on BJ's previous stress-reduction skills and past experiences, if any, with anxiety.

4. *What management options would you recommend?*

   Our clinic's intervention protocol for tinnitus includes the Jastreboff Tinnitus Retraining Therapy (TRT) program and for hyperacusis the Jastreboff desensitization protocol. Typically, we recommend completion of the first 3-week desensitization protocol before employing sound therapy, but due to BJ's severe lifestyle limitations and concomitant tinnitus, both approaches were implemented simultaneously. In most cases, completion of the desensitization protocol should increase the patient's dynamic range and allow them to employ sound therapy as needed for tinnitus. Because BJ expressed all sounds were too loud, the clinicians decided the best management approach was to use the two protocols together.

5. *What medical professional(s) would you recommend her to see?*

   Due to her sleep disturbances, difficult eating, and reported symptoms of anxiety, BJ should be seen by her primary care physician, a mental health professional, and potentially a dietitian. Many of her difficulties fall outside the scope of audiology, and although they may be related to her audiologic problems, it is important she seek care from other health care professionals. An interdisciplinary treatment approach for this patient is most optimal.

19.6 Recommendations and Outcomes

BJ's case history, initial interview, and tinnitus evaluation revealed significant sound intolerance and severe bilateral tinnitus. In addition, BJ's reports of difficulty eating, sleeping, and touching her face/hair/ears indicate referral to determine the possibility of co-occurring anxiety. The clinicians carefully explained the tinnitus/hyperacusis cycle and management options. BJ expressed confusion regarding her diagnosis of hyperacusis, stating she thought hyperacusis was a low-level hearing loss caused by anxiety. We explained the difference between hyperacusis and hearing loss, as well as explained how patients with tinnitus and sound sensitivities often also experience anxiety.

Our main priority for management for BJ was to reduce the use of ear protection in quiet and to minimize her avoidance of sounds. We recommended BJ complete desensitization exercises to help manage her hyperacusis, which she was willing to try. We also recommended she employ the use of sound therapy through a phone app to replace ear protection, with the intent of fostering tinnitus habituation. BJ was hesitant to employ sound therapy, as she perceived all sounds offered by various apps as "too fast" or "too busy." Instead of beginning with the desensitization protocol and later moving into sound therapy, we adapted the management approach and used the two protocols together. In addition, we recommended she enroll in and complete the Mindfulness Tinnitus Stress Reduction Course, offered free during the pandemic quarantine by Jennifer Gans, PhD. Mindfulness-based tinnitus stress reduction techniques may reduce tinnitus severity as indicated by improved TFI and THI scores within 4 weeks.[5] The tinnitus cycle (the neurophysiologic model of tinnitus) explains the central perception of a signal generated in the auditory system where the perception results in annoyance of the listener, which causes the listener to focus more on the signal and exacerbates the annoyance in a cyclical fashion.[6] Mindfulness-based practices likely reduce perceived stress associated with tinnitus because it helps to interrupt the negative tinnitus cycle, thus potentially reducing limbic system responses.

BJ communicated with the clinicians via email for several weeks following her evaluation. She reported initial relief from utilizing sound therapy in place of ear protection and noise avoidance, but noted persistent sleeping difficulties. About a week later, BJ reported her hyperacusis, reactive tinnitus, anxiety, and emotional distress to have worsened exponentially. She reported new, explicit fear of sounds as minute as the air conditioner. In addition, she reported a numbing and tingling sensation in her face accompanying the presence of offensive sounds and anxiety. BJ indicated she understood her condition to be related to her lymphatic system instead of her limbic system, which had been described by the clinicians at the time of her initial testing. BJ was given additional information about the potential for tinnitus to produce a negative cycle of distress and intrusiveness. The clinicians advised BJ she may now be experiencing phonophobia, or fear hyperacusis. BJ was encouraged to meet with her physician regarding the tingling sensation and to schedule an appointment with a mental health professional to discuss her sound sensitivity and anxiety.

19.7 Self-Efficacy Considerations for the Clinician

- Patients with tinnitus and fear hyperacusis often exhibit comorbid psychological conditions. Be aware of signs of anxiety, depression, and maladaptive thought processes in your patients, and take care to modify counseling and management recommendations as appropriate. A referral network is essential with these patients. Many psychology professionals are unaware of sound sensitivity disorders and are ill-equipped to treat them. Finding an appropriate referral network is time well spent.
- Patients may misunderstand diagnoses and may self-educate on their perceived diagnosis. It is important to thoroughly counsel patients regarding their diagnosis and make appropriate recommendations. This may take several attempts of reframing the explanation of diagnosis and educating the patient on our management recommendations. In addition,

clinicians should feel confident modifying test protocol (i.e., omitting immittance testing) in cases of reactive tinnitus and hyperacusis to best fit the patients' needs.

References

[1] Locke A, Kirst N, Shultz C. Diagnosis and management of generalized anxiety disorder and panic disorder in adults; 2015. Retrieved August 4, 2020, from https://www.aafp.org/afp/2015/0501/p617.html

[2] Meikle MB, Henry JA, Griest SE, et al. The Tinnitus Functional Index: development of a new clinical measure for chronic, intrusive tinnitus. Ear Hear. 2012; 33(2):153–176

[3] Newman CW, Jacobson GP, Spitzer JB. Development of the Tinnitus Handicap Inventory. Arch Otolaryngol Head Neck Surg. 1996; 122(2):143–148

[4] Sawamoto N, Honda M, Okada T, et al. Expectation of pain enhances responses to nonpainful somatosensory stimulation in the anterior cingulate cortex and parietal operculum/posterior insula: an event-related functional magnetic resonance imaging study; 2000. Retrieved August 4, 2020, from https://www.jneurosci.org/content/20/19/7438

[5] Roland LT, Lenze EJ, Hardin F, et al. Effects of mindfulness based stress reduction therapy on subjective bother and neural connectivity in chronic tinnitus; 2015. Retrieved from https://pubmed.ncbi.nlm.nih.gov//25715350/

[6] Jastreboff PJ, Hazell JW, Graham RL. Neurophysiological model of tinnitus: dependence of the minimal masking level on treatment outcome. Hear Res. 1994 Nov;80(2):216-232. doi: 10.1016/0378-5955(94)90113-9

Suggested Reading

Henry JA, Jastreboff MM, Jastreboff PJ, Schechter MA, Fausti SA. Guide to conducting tinnitus retraining therapy initial and follow-up interviews. J Rehabil Res Dev. 2003; 40(2):157–177

20 Tinnitus and Hyponatremia

Christopher Kuykendall and Suzanne H. Kimball

20.1 Clinical History and Description

NM, a 35-year-old female immigrant from Central Asia, was seen at a University Speech and Hearing Clinic with the chief complaint of right unilateral tinnitus. Case history indicated history of anxiety and a recent diagnosis of right unilateral high frequency hearing loss. She reported that she first heard her tinnitus on June 6, 2018 while bending over, describing the tinnitus as sounding like crickets at onset, changing over time to a waterfall sound. Prior to this date's evaluation, she reported consuming a portion of a Mucinex (over-the-counter) decongestion pill. Subsequently, she read on the Internet that taking a partial pill could be toxic. NM became very anxious about the potential negative effects of having taken the pill, and decided to "flush" her system by drinking more than 70 bottles of water over a short amount of time. This action ultimately resulted in NM being admitted to an Intensive Care Unit (ICU) for multiple days due to hyponatremia, or an abnormally low concentration of sodium in her blood.

20.2 Audiological Testing

NM initially received a comprehensive audiologic examination at an ENT and Audiology hospital clinic. This examination revealed normal hearing sensitivity through 4,000 Hz steeply sloping to a moderate-to-severe hearing loss at 6,000 and 8,000 Hz for the right ear and normal hearing sensitivity for the left ear from 250 to 8,000 Hz with a negative pure-tone Stenger (see ▶ Fig. 20.1). Her pure-tone average (PTA) was 8 dB HL for the right ear and 5 dB HL for the left ear. The tympanometric results, including ear canal volume, static admittance, and middle ear pressure were all within the normal range bilaterally. Acoustic reflex thresholds (ARTs) were absent in the left contralateral condition, present in the right contralateral condition, and present in both ipsilateral conditions. The SRT of 5 dB HL in each ear was consistent with the PTA, and the word recognition score in quiet was excellent bilaterally with negative performance intensity-phonetically balanced (PI-PB) rollover at 80 dB HL for the right ear and at 85 dB HL for the left ear (▶ Fig. 20.1). This evaluation was followed by an ENT consultation conducted by a Physicians Associate (PA). The PA concluded NM's tinnitus was likely related to a sudden hearing loss in her right ear. The PA then referred NM to our clinic for a tinnitus evaluation, recommended a round of steroids to treat the unilateral hearing loss, and recommended a magnetic resonance imaging (MRI) regarding the asymmetric hearing loss and tinnitus to rule out the rare possibility of a benign tumor on NM's vestibulocochlear nerve. While at our clinic, NM reported she was not interested in receiving the MRI due to her concern about the gadolinium contrast with which she would be injected during the examination.

20.3 Questions for the Reader

1. Is it uncommon for those who are experiencing a sudden hearing loss to struggle with anxiety?
2. What is hyponatremia and why is it important for this case?

20.4 Discussion of Questions for the Reader

1. *Is it uncommon for those who are experiencing a sudden hearing loss to struggle with anxiety?*
   No. Many people who experience a sudden hearing loss with bothersome tinnitus also are highly anxious.[1] We noted anxiety in NM, supported by the report of her response to consuming a partial Mucinex pill, and her reservations about gadolinium contrast that compelled her to decline the recommended MRI.
2. *What is hyponatremia and why is it important for this case?*
   Hyponatremia is a very rare depletion of sodium (K) in the blood. In this case, it was caused by the over consumption of water in a very short time. When sodium levels become too low, liquid, primarily water, is driven by forces of equilibrium and diffuses from one's blood and tissues to inside their cells via osmosis, causing the cells to swell and in extreme cases, break apart. This presents a potentially fatal circumstance when the cells in the brain begin to swell.

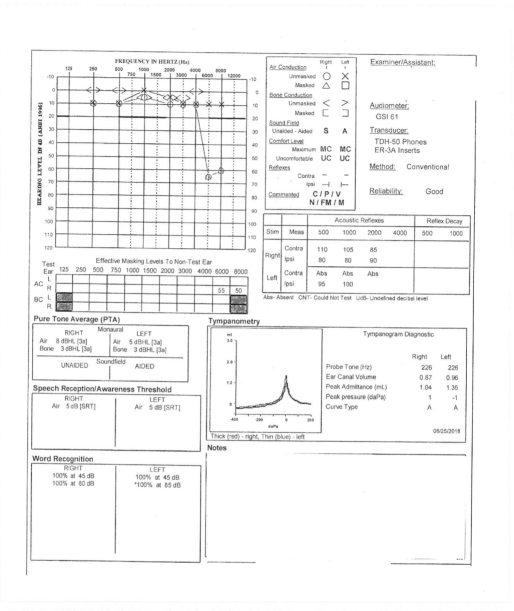

Fig. 20.1 Initial hearing evaluation performed at local otolaryngology practice.

20.5 Tinnitus Evaluation

Additional testing took place at our clinic approximately 2 months after her initial hearing evaluation at the ENT audiology hospital clinic. Otoscopy revealed nonoccluding cerumen bilaterally.

a) Ultra high-frequency audiometry revealed that the aforementioned moderate-to-severe hearing loss continued through 16,000 Hz before rising to normal hearing sensitivity from 18,000 to 20,000 Hz for the right ear and normal hearing sensitivity in the left ear from 10,000 to 20,000 Hz with the exception of a response in the mild range at 16,000 Hz for the left ear (see ▶ Fig. 20.2).

b) A tinnitus evaluation was conducted for the right ear and revealed the following: pitch match (1,000 Hz), loudness match (10 dB SL re: pure-tone threshold at 1,000 Hz for the right ear), minimum masking level for white noise (10 dB SL re: white noise threshold for the right ear), and

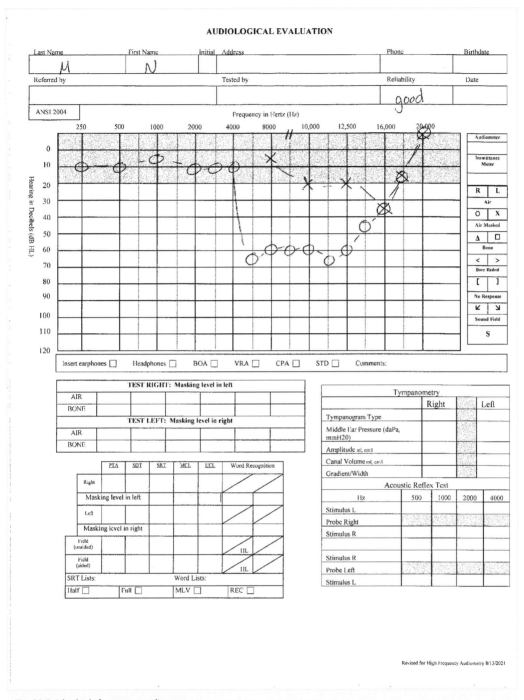

Fig. 20.2 Ultrahigh-frequency audiogram.

residual inhibition (no change in tinnitus perception).

c) Scores and answers for the Tinnitus Handicap Inventory (THI) and the Tinnitus Functional Index (TFI) were obtained. THI score was 26 and TFI score was 20. These results indicated that NM was mildly bothered by her tinnitus.

20.6 Additional Questions for the Reader

1. Based on her history and audiometric results, what differential diagnoses should be considered?
2. What types of audiologic intervention would be appropriate?
3. What additional test(s) could be recommended?

20.7 Discussion of Additional Questions for the Reader

1. *Based on her history and audiometric results, what differential diagnoses should be considered?*
   a) Sudden unilateral hearing loss: One of the primary sources of tinnitus is damage to the auditory system. Due to NM's report of sudden unilateral tinnitus and the finding of a previously unperceived unilateral hearing loss, it could be that her tinnitus was associated with a sudden hearing loss in her right ear that she did not notice upon its sudden onset.
   b) Acoustic neuroma: Unilateral hearing loss as confirmed by conventional pure-tone and ultra high-frequency pure-tone testing along with unilateral tinnitus are certainly red flags for an acoustic neuroma. However, a suspected right side acoustic neuroma would most likely be accompanied by elevated or absent right ipsilateral and contralateral acoustic reflexes and with poorer than expected or asymmetric word recognition scores with positive rollover.
   c) Central lesion: Elevated or absent contralateral acoustic reflexes along with present or mildly elevated ipsilateral reflexes are the primary red flag for a central lesion, specifically the intra-axial brainstem. Further, with NM's history, it could be possible that she obtained damage to her brainstem related to the swelling that accompanies hyponatremia. This swelling could be in such an area that it only affected NM's right auditory system.
2. *What types of audiologic intervention would be appropriate?*
   a) This clinic's primary intervention for bothersome tinnitus includes amplification if a hearing loss is present and sound therapy. When this clinic utilizes sound therapy, we establish the optimal masker level by finding each patient's "mixing point," which we determine by reducing the masker output slightly from the point at which the stimulus completely masks the tinnitus. The patient is informed that the sound therapy should be utilized at a level softer than the level producing complete masking, resulting in a masker level that allows the tinnitus to be barely perceptible. Typically, this level is 6 to 13 dB HL lower than the so-called "mixing point." We recommend utilizing sound therapy at this level so that the masker can interact with the tinnitus without making it inaudible. This protocol is intended to foster habituation of the tinnitus sound. Please note that the masker should never be set to a level that is uncomfortable for the patient, even if the masker level follows the general rule indicated above.
   b) With the recent developments in hearing aids, monaural amplification could provide gain in the high and ultra-high-frequency ranges. However, because NM does not perceive a hearing loss in her right ear, the main advantage of the hearing aid would be to amplify environmental sounds that can contribute to tinnitus masking. Tinnitus Retraining Therapy (TRT), the tinnitus rehabilitation program used in this clinic, strongly recommends the patient receive sound therapy binaurally; hearing aids would be costly in this case as she has a unilateral loss that does not produce functional difficulties.
   c) Sound therapy is delivered through an app on her smart phone or tablet. Sound therapy is readily available at no cost through applications developed by most hearing aid manufacturers and can be downloaded easily through the Apple App Store or Google Play.
3. *What additional test(s) could be recommended?*
   A diagnostic auditory brainstem response (ABR) would offer a logical next test for this patient. If the ABR showed any abnormalities, an MRI test could be completed. These diagnostic tests may be required to definitively identify the cause of her auditory symptoms.
   The American Academy of Otolaryngology-Head and Neck Surgery recommends not using an imaging study to evaluate bilateral tinnitus. This case is unique because although the patient's chief complaint was unilateral tinnitus, many other concerns were revealed that could potentially warrant an MRI study.

20.8 Final Diagnosis and Recommended Treatment

NM's hearing and tinnitus evaluations revealed unilateral hearing loss in the high and ultra-high frequencies, mild unilateral tinnitus, and abnormal contralateral acoustic reflexes. NM seemed to be experiencing difficulties that could potentially be due to anxiety and complications from hyponatremia. To address her anxiety, we recommended psychiatric counseling and care. We strongly recommended that NM undergo an ABR and potentially an MRI to explore possible pathologies that could be secondary to hyponatremia. We further recommended the use of sound therapy through an app to manage her tinnitus.

20.9 Outcome

It was reported by NM's husband approximately 6 months after our evaluation that her symptoms had not changed. He further explained that she has taken the initiative to read some literature (uncited) about tinnitus and hearing loss and is no longer concerned about her symptoms. Because she has noticed no additional changes in her symptoms, she has made the decision not to seek any further testing or treatment.

20.10 Self-Efficacy for the Clinician

- Patients who experience bothersome tinnitus are often also anxious, which can lead to unique challenges for the patient and clinician, and can complicate management and recommendations.

- Acoustic reflexes offer valuable information regarding potential site of lesion.
- A thorough audiologic evaluation is imperative regardless of what the patient presents as their chief complaint.
- There are many causes of tinnitus, which makes it very important to approach each patient without preconceived notions as well as to be diligent to details of medical history.
- We live in an age that allows the individuals we are helping to self-educate. It is our job to make the appropriate recommendations regardless of what they read. It is ultimately up to the patient to decide what they will do.

References

[1] Pattyn T, Van Den Eede F, Vanneste S, et al. Tinnitus and anxiety disorders: a review. Hear Res. 2016; 333:255–265

[2] Newman CW, Jacobson GP, Spitzer JB. Development of the Tinnitus Handicap Inventory. Arch Otolaryngol Head Neck Surg. 1996; 122(2):143–148

[3] Meikle MB, Henry JA, Griest SE, et al. The tinnitus functional index: development of a new clinical measure for chronic, intrusive tinnitus. Ear Hear. 2012; 33(2):153–176

Suggested Readings

Shargorodsky J, Curhan GC, Farwell WR. Prevalence and characteristics of tinnitus among US adults. Am J Med. 2010; 123(8):711–718

Adrogué HJ, Madias NE. Hyponatremia. N Engl J Med. 2000; 342 (21):1581–1589

Jerger S, Jerger J. Diagnostic value of crossed vs uncrossed acoustic reflexes: eighth nerve and brain stem disorders. Arch Otolaryngol. 1977; 103(8):445–453

Kehrle HM, Sampaio AL, Granjeiro RC, de Oliveira TS, Oliveira CA. Tinnitus annoyance in normal-hearing individuals: Correlation with depression and anxiety. Ann Otol Rhinol Laryngol. 2016; 125(3):185–194

Tunkel DE, Bauer CA, Sun GH, et al. Clinical practice guideline: tinnitus. Otolaryngol Head Neck Surg. 2014; 151(2) Suppl:S1–S40

21 "Ellie": Psychological Management of Tinnitus in the Context of Pediatric OCD

Myles S. Rizvi

21.1 Clinical History and Description

Ellie is a 10-year-old girl who was referred to our clinic for obsessive-compulsive disorder (OCD) and health-related anxiety. Ellie reported recurrent and intrusive fears about having illnesses or diseases. Her fear triggers included touching tall grass and dirt (for fear of contracting Lyme disease), hearing others talk about medical conditions, and being in hospitals in the presence of children her age who appeared ill (e.g., wearing hospital gowns). Physical symptoms (e.g., headaches, dizziness) also triggered Ellie's fears of illness, at which time she often worried about what these symptoms might mean medically (for example, she expressed concern regarding possible meningitis). A noteworthy trigger to Ellie's fears of illness included ear ringing associated with tinnitus, where she similarly worried about what ear ringing might indicate (e.g., stroke). Ellie often sought reassurance from her parents for example, asking them to check her temperature, in order to address her concerns, and the family admitted to having difficulty with consoling Ellie and convincing her that she was not seriously ill.

21.2 Audiologic Testing

Ellie completed an audiological diagnostic assessment in September 2018 to evaluate her ear ringing, which reportedly began in December 2017. Ellie and her family described her ear ringing as infrequent, noting that stress triggered her tinnitus and headaches. She indicated that her tinnitus was most bothersome at night when she tried to fall asleep; the family reported using a white noise machine to facilitate sleep. Ellie denied experiencing tinnitus and headaches simultaneously. The family denied a history of ear infections or ear pain/fullness. According to the audiological diagnostic evaluation, conventional audiometry carried out under circumaural headphones revealed a speech recognition threshold of 5 dB HL, bilaterally, and reliable responses to pure-tone air-conducted stimuli were obtained in the normal range for both ears. Tympanometry revealed normal, type A, tympanograms bilaterally, consistent with normal middle ear function. Acoustic reflexes could not be assessed due to the patient's reported anxiety regarding the test. Ellie reported that she was worried about being confined in the testing room rather than the test itself, expressing that she experiences anxiety when in enclosed spaces (e.g., elevators). Distortion-product otoacoustic emissions were present for both ears, consistent with normal outer hair cell function bilaterally.

21.3 Questions for the Reader

1. What thoughts and behaviors did Ellie exhibit and were recapitulated by her family that maintained her fears, distress, and tinnitus-related anxiety?
2. Why might conventional coping skills (e.g., diaphragmatic breathing, distraction) for tinnitus be contraindicated in Ellie's case?
3. Exposure-based interventions, where the patient systematically approaches fear triggers without engaging in avoidance behavior, are empirically supported treatments for OCD and anxiety. How should exposure-based interventions be applied to tinnitus-related anxiety and distress?

21.4 Discussion of Questions for the Reader

1. *What thoughts and behaviors did Ellie exhibit and were recapitulated by her family that maintain her fears, distress, and tinnitus-related anxiety?*

   Overestimation of threat and intolerance of uncertainty reportedly underlie and sustain obsessions and repetitive safety behaviors (i.e., compulsions) in adult[1] and pediatric cases of OCD.[2] According to the fear-avoidance model for chronic tinnitus,[3,4,5,6] individuals may misinterpret ear ringing as harmful or threatening, resulting in tinnitus-related fear. The fear response may provoke avoidance and escape behaviors that over time become negatively reinforced through immediate short-term relief. Unfortunately, long-term avoidance of tinnitus triggers and tinnitus itself maintains the heightened fear response. In turn, the high-threat expectancies and tinnitus-related fear may increase tinnitus severity and distress.[7] As with many other patients, Ellie overestimated the threat posed by her tinnitus. Ellie's interpretation of tinnitus as dangerous also manifested in her uncertainty as to what tinnitus might signify medically. Ellie was uncomfortable about not knowing why her ears ring and she avoided this distress by repeatedly checking with her parents in an attempt to "know," akin to an individual with OCD who frequently checks the locks to confirm they are indeed locked. Ellie's reassurance seeking provided short-term relief while inadvertently teaching Ellie that the only way for her to tolerate the distress of uncertainty was by avoiding it entirely, thus reinforcing her distress and commensurate avoidance behaviors. Her family's assurance that she is healthy and not likely to develop feared illnesses, although well intentioned, reinforced Ellie's anxiety regarding uncertainty.

2. *Why might conventional coping skills (e.g., diaphragmatic breathing, distraction) for tinnitus be contraindicated in Ellie's case?*
Individuals with OCD typically engage in avoidance to reduce distress caused by obsessions, not only by engaging in compulsions and avoiding environmental triggers but also by avoiding distressing thoughts and sensory experiences. Thought suppression (e.g., deliberately avoiding thinking about the challenging condition or environment) and distraction (e.g., thinking about something else) are common strategies used to avoid thoughts and sensations. Research demonstrated that attempts to suppress thoughts were associated with increases in thought frequency[8] and that attempts to suppress emotion were associated with higher negative emotional intensity[9] and anxiety.[10] Conventional self-regulation strategies, such as diaphragmatic breathing, may inadvertently reinforce beliefs that physical sensations are dangerous. Engaging in these strategies may prevent the individual from learning that sensory experiences like tinnitus (as unpleasant and uncomfortable as they may be) are not dangerous and, perhaps most importantly, can be tolerated. Effective emotion management requires a degree of acceptance and tolerance of unpleasant emotional experiences, and efforts to distract from or downregulate emotional or sensory experiences (i.e., tinnitus) prevent improvements in distress tolerance.

3. *Exposure-based interventions, where the patient systematically approaches fear triggers without engaging in avoidance behavior, are empirically supported treatments for OCD and anxiety. How should exposure-based interventions be applied to tinnitus-related anxiety and distress?*
Many patients with severe tinnitus exhibit obsessive thoughts or compulsive behaviors related to their auditory symptoms,[11] often being anxious about personal health issues and engaging in compulsions by repeatedly checking the status of their tinnitus or environmental sound levels, which prevent them from getting used to (i.e., habituating) their tinnitus. Therefore, exposure-based interventions would involve having patients systematically expose themselves to these triggers without engaging in compulsive and/or avoidant behavior. Regarding the experience of tinnitus itself, patients would be counseled regarding tinnitus mechanisms, its lack of threat, and instructed to attend to the tinnitus (rather than distracting themselves from it) to facilitate tolerance and eventual habituation.

21.5 Final Diagnosis and Recommended Treatment

Ellie's diagnosis of OCD, wherein her intrusive health-related fears were framed as obsessions and her reassurance-seeking behaviors viewed as checking compulsions conducted to reduce these fears. Ellie's health-related fears extended to her tinnitus, and it became apparent throughout treatment that she additionally worried that ear ringing, when experienced, would "not go away." It was recommended that Ellie and her parents participate in cognitive-behavioral therapy (CBT) involving exposure-based interventions. The family was educated on the cycle of anxiety, avoidance, and accommodation, namely that Ellie's avoidance of fear triggers (including physical sensations like tinnitus) and reassurance-seeking behaviors were maintaining her fears. The importance of decreasing avoidance and family accommodation was discussed with the family, and ways in which the family could respond to Ellie's reassurance seeking without accommodating the behavior were modeled and role-played.

Ellie's fear triggers were collaboratively listed and hierarchically arranged by having Ellie use a numerical system to rate her distress resulting from each fear trigger. Among her list of fear triggers were physical feelings, including headaches, tinnitus, muscle aches, and dizziness. Interoceptive exposure therapy, which involves purposefully inducing physical symptoms of anxiety, was introduced as a way in which Ellie could get used to these physical sensations and learn they were not dangerous and intolerable. Ellie first completed interoceptive exposures designed to simulate dizziness, including taking hyperventilating breaths and spinning in an office chair. Ellie became progressive less distressed by these exercises, and she subsequently completed interoceptive exposures simulating tinnitus, including mimicking her ear-ringing sound and listening to ear-ring sounds on YouTube. After she similarly habituated to these exercises, Ellie agreed to complete exposure exercises requiring her to practice thinking feared thoughts (e.g., she might have an illness) and refrain from engaging reassurance seeking and other compulsions (e.g., tapping foot five times to prevent illness).

21.6 Outcome

As tinnitus-related exposures became easier for Ellie to complete, subsequent exposures involved using more anxiety-provoking YouTube videos involving dramatic warning signs (e.g., needing to see an ear specialist after listening to the video); Ellie also tolerated these exercises well. Ellie was praised for her participation in exposures, and she was asked what she learned from her practice, to which she related that she learned that she "got used to" anxiety, physical feelings, and tinnitus, noting that these sensations went away on their own. On the eighth outpatient therapy session, Ellie denied experiencing tinnitus and associated worries. Her father concurrently indicated that Ellie has not complained or exhibited worry about tinnitus, adding that she has been using her white noise machine less. Ellie was told that ear ringing, for whatever reason, may return, and that should this happen, she should be able to understand it and tolerate it more easily than in the past.

References

[1] Grøtte T, Solem S, Myers SG, et al. Metacognitions in obsessive-compulsive disorder: a psychometric study of the Metacognitions Questionnaire-30. J Obsessive Compuls Relat Disord. 2016; 11:82–90

[2] Schultz C, Lambek R, Højgaard D, et al. Psychometric validation of a Danish version of the Obsessive Beliefs Questionnaire–Child Version (OBQ-CV). Nord J Psychiatry. 2018; 72(8):621–629 Advance online publication

[3] Cima RFF, Crombez G, Vlaeyen JWS. Catastrophizing and fear of tinnitus predict quality of life in patients with chronic tinnitus. Ear Hear. 2011; 32(5):634–641

[4] Hallam RS, Rachman S, Hinchcliffe R. Psychological aspects of tinnitus. In: Rachman S, ed. Contributions to medical psychology, Vol. 3. Oxford: Pergamon Press; 1984

[5] Kleinstäuber M, Jasper K, Schweda I, Hiller W, Andersson G, Weise C. The role of fear-avoidance cognitions and behaviors in patients with chronic tinnitus. Cogn Behav Ther. 2013; 42 (2):84–99

[6] McKenna L, Handscomb L, Hoare DJ, Hall DA. A scientific cognitive-behavioral model of tinnitus: novel conceptualizations of tinnitus distress. Front Neurol. 2014; 5:196

[7] Cima RFF, van Breukelen G, Vlaeyen JWS. Tinnitus-related fear: mediating the effects of a cognitive behavioural specialised tinnitus treatment. Hear Res. 2018; 358:86–97

[8] Abramowitz JS, Tolin DF, Street GP. Paradoxical effects of thought suppression: a meta-analysis of controlled studies. Clin Psychol Rev. 2001; 21(5):683–703

[9] Lynch TA, Robins CJ, Morse JO, Krause ED. A mediational model relating affect intensity, emotional inhibition, and psychological distress. Behav Ther. 2001; 32:519–536

[10] Levitt JT, Brown TA, Orsillo SM, Barlow DH. The effects of acceptance versus suppression of emotion on subjective and psychophysiological response to carbon dioxide challenge in patients with panic disorder. Behav Ther. 2004; 35:747–766

[11] Folmer RL, Griest SE, Martin WH. Obsessive-compulsiveness in a population of tinnitus patients. Int Tinnitus J. 2008; 14 (2):127–130

22 Psychogenic Tinnitus and Dizziness

Suzanne H. Kimball and Christi Barbee

22.1 Case History and Description

LG, a 42-year-old female, self-referred to our clinic for a hearing evaluation due to difficulty understanding conversations with her family and at work. LG is employed as a part-time crisis intervention specialist. Due to her initial complaints, LG was scheduled for three separate appointments: a comprehensive audiometric evaluation, a tinnitus evaluation, and a vestibular evaluation. She was also later scheduled for a hearing aid fitting. Each session will be discussed separately.

22.2 Audiologic Evaluation

On her initial evaluation, LG reported that she "got into trouble" at work due to the volume of her voice while on the phone. She further reported difficulty maintaining an appropriate vocal volume in daily living and in situations with significant background noise. LG reported all of the following at her initial evaluation: (1) hearing loss which appeared to be worse in her left ear; (2) long-standing, severe, constant tinnitus, which more recently had made her nauseous and dizzy; (3) sound sensitivity to static and loud noises, which also induced nausea; (4) foot pain while walking; (5) cold feet; (6) a body that felt like it was being "squeezed" constantly; and (7) bilateral aural "discomfort." Lastly, LG reported issues with word retrieval and memory.

22.3 Test Results

Acoustic immittance testing identified a type A tympanogram for the left ear. A tympanogram could not be obtained for the right ear due to aural discomfort. Acoustic reflex thresholds could not be obtained due to patient concern regarding the anticipated sound levels. Pure-tone testing indicated a mild-to-moderate high-frequency sensorineural hearing loss bilaterally. Speech recognition thresholds (SRT) were established at 30 dB HL for both ears and were in good agreement with pure-tone averages indicating good reliability. Word recognition scores (WRS) were 88% for the right ear and 80% for the left ear, presented at 55 dB HL in quiet (see audiogram in ▶ Fig. 22.1). Recommendations

from this testing included: (1) follow-up with primary care physician regarding global health concerns, (2) tinnitus evaluation, (3) vestibular evaluation, (4) binaural amplification, and (5) referral to Disability Resource Services (DRS) to provide workplace accommodations and financial assistance.

22.4 Questions for the Reader; Audiologic Evaluation

1. Of the intake information and audiologic test results, which indicate aspects of the case that must be addressed by a clinician focused on tinnitus assessment and management?
2. Of the intake information and audiologic test results, which indicate aspects of the case that must be addressed by a clinician focused on vestibular assessment and management?

22.5 Discussion of Questions for the Reader; Audiologic Evaluation

1. *Of the intake information and audiologic test results, which indicate aspects of the case that must be addressed by a clinician focused on tinnitus assessment and management?*
   Based on the patient's initial complaints, the clinician should focus on tinnitus management, and expand the case history to include elements associated with tinnitus intrusiveness. Loudness tolerance testing, if employed, must be implemented with caution to minimize dizziness or nausea.
2. *Of the intake information and audiologic test results, which indicate aspects of the case that must be addressed by a clinician focused on vestibular assessment and management?*
   Due to this patient's reported global health concerns, as part of a thorough case history, the clinician involved in vestibular assessment should document a detailed description of movements or actions that provoke the sensation of vertigo, as well as the patient's medications, including those that are over the counter (OTC) to determine any possible contraindications for balance issues.

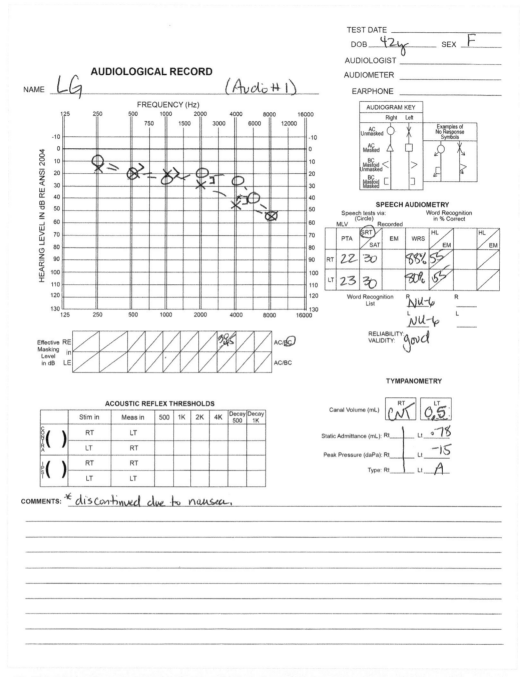

Fig. 22.1 Initial audiogram obtained indicating mild-to-moderate high-frequency sensorineural hearing loss.

22.6 Tinnitus Evaluation

LG returned for her tinnitus evaluation approximately 1 week after her first visit to our clinic. She presented to this appointment visibly shaken and highly distracted. She revealed that in the days just prior to the appointment, she experienced a traumatic event in which her own daughter threatened her life by attempting to stab her. LG indicated that her hearing loss played a role in her safety in this situation because she was unable to hear the approaching threat and had to rely on a family member to save her life. Once the patient calmed down a bit in the testing suite, we were able to move forward with the evaluation.

At this appointment, LG reported severe sensitivity to loud sounds, which had profoundly affected her quality of life, as well as tinnitus that was exacerbated by stress and anxiety. LG's symptoms were reported as much more severe since her daughter had threatened her. LG also revealed that she was being seen by a behavioral therapist and treated by a chiropractor for her tinnitus. She reported additional tinnitus interventions including essential oils, OTC anxiety medications, and jawline massaging.

22.7 Tinnitus Evaluation Test Results

High-frequency audiometry and uncomfortable loudness testing were conducted. High-frequency audiometry revealed a moderate to moderately-severe hearing loss bilaterally from 9,000 to 20,000 Hz. Uncomfortable loudness testing identified severely reduced loudness tolerance levels for both speech and pure-tone conditions (65–75 dB HL) (see audiogram in ▶ Fig. 22.2). The tinnitus evaluation could not be completed as LG could not tolerate testing procedures, and in addition, she declined to complete her questionnaires. Recommendations from this appointment included addressing the extreme sound intolerance before considering amplification, and to that end, she was provided desensitization exercises. She was advised to continue to work with her therapist to address anxiety that reportedly worsened her reaction to tinnitus and sound sensitivity symptoms.

22.8 Questions for the Reader; Tinnitus Evaluation

1. Is it uncommon for those with tinnitus and extreme sound intolerance to have high levels of anxiety?
2. What concerns do the sound intolerance present regarding hearing aid usage?

22.9 Discussion of Questions for the Reader: Tinnitus Evaluation

1. *Is it uncommon for those with tinnitus and extreme sound intolerance to have high levels of anxiety?*

No. Anxiety is by far one of the most common comorbidities of tinnitus and sound intolerance. Granted, this patient had an extreme case of anxiety, which was brought on by a life stressor unfamiliar to most patients (e.g., being attacked by one's own daughter). This likely played a role in her testing, response to intervention, and outcomes.

2. *What concerns do the sound intolerance present regarding hearing aid usage?*

Amplification may cause a patient to perceive sounds to be "too loud" in general, and as a result, decline device use. For someone with extreme sound intolerance (likely fear or loudness hyperacusis in this case,[1] amplification may be difficult to accept, and could potentially make the situation worse. Desensitization is a well-established approach to facilitating exposure to sensory events that otherwise have the potential to produce discomfort.

22.10 Balance Assessment

The patient returned to our clinic about 6 weeks later for a vestibular assessment intended to investigate her chief complaint of increasing difficulty with balance. She reported becoming symptomatic when turning her head and when getting out of bed. She reported needing to hold onto a family member to maintain balance while walking. She reported that her prescription glasses made her dizzy and that she experienced diplopia (seeing two images as a single object) 1 week prior to this evaluation. She said her balance issues worsened when her tinnitus symptoms increased. She was unable to identify exactly when her balance troubles began, but she indicated that over the past several years her symptoms continued to worsen. She saw a chiropractor for treatment, but due to financial considerations had to discontinue that intervention. LG's medication list included Naturethroid (OTC), Vitamin B12, Vitamin D/Calcium, Omega 3 Fish Oil, Magnesium, Zinc, and Biotin. Aside from the diplopia, she reported numerous falls, bilateral otalgia, tinnitus, headaches, dizziness, nausea, anxiety/depression, intermittent vertigo lasting seconds to minutes, transient numbness, and tingling in the leg and foot. Her Dizziness Handicap Inventory Score was a 54, indicating a severe handicap.[2] vHIT testing revealed responses, but had to be aborted because LG became quickly nauseous. Further testing could not be completed. A neurological evaluation was recommended.

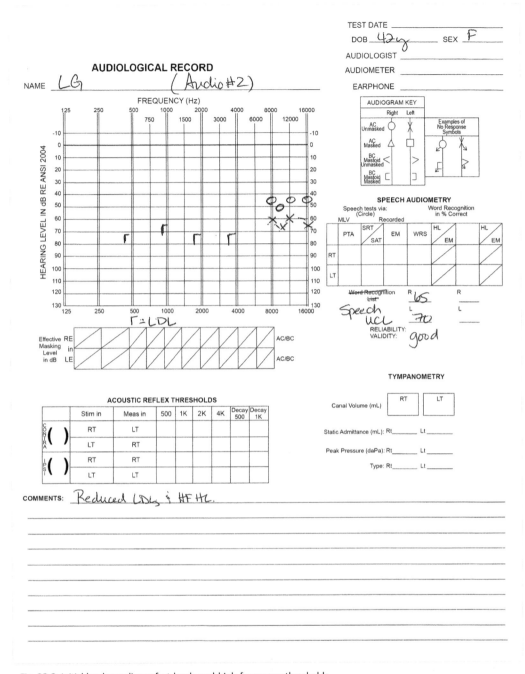

Fig. 22.2 Initial loudness discomfort levels and high frequency thresholds.

22.11 Questions for the Reader; Vestibular Evaluation

1. Is it uncommon for those with dizziness to suffer from high levels of anxiety?

2. Do OTC medications or supplements affect balance and dizziness?

22.12 Discussion of Questions to the Reader; Vestibular Evaluation

1. *Is it uncommon for those with dizziness to suffer from high levels of anxiety?*
   No. Anxiety is common in patients who experience dizziness. Dizziness may create the sensation of being out of control. LG displayed symptoms of anxiety and possibly of neurologic disease. Either anxiety or neurologic disease may cause a patient to have dizziness. As LG would not allow a complete vestibular evaluation, inner ear contribution could not be fully ruled out; however, a neurologic consult was recommended.
2. *Do OTC medications or supplements affect balance and dizziness?*
   Yes. OTC medications or supplements may affect balance. In this case, LG was relying on supplements and OTC medications as she felt this was a safer option than prescription medication. Reviewing all medications including supplements and OTC medications is necessary as OTC treatment may change prescription medication effectiveness. A pharmacist should be recruited to review the combination of medications and supplements to identify potential negative interactions.

22.13 Common Features to all Appointments

Since all three appointments were conducted within the same center, the first author had the advantage of visiting with all of the providers in this case. Common to each of the appointments was LG's pattern of clinical reporting and testing. At each appointment, LG presented her symptoms and experiences in a manner similar to a "chaos narrative" in which she spoke in disjointed, poorly organized phrases during her intake interviews to describe a litany of wide-ranging symptoms. Each symptom's association to hearing loss, tinnitus, sound intolerance, or balance issues was difficult to assess, and clearly a source of confusion for the patient. She often got "off topic," did not, or could not answer questions directly, often seemed distracted, and was vague in most answers when directly questioned. This made determining an appropriate course of action for her quite challenging.

Despite the inconsistencies and uncertainty, audiologic rehabilitation was deemed a reasonable starting point for intervention.

22.14 Hearing Aid Fitting

Repeated test results confirmed a mild sloping to moderate high-frequency sensorineural hearing loss. LG was fitted with binaural receiver-in-the-canal (RIC) hearing aids 6 weeks after her tinnitus evaluation, and on the same day as her vestibular evaluation. Prior to the fitting, loudness discomfort measures were repeated (see audiogram #3 in ▶ Fig. 22.3). All measures were found to be within normal limits on this date. LG indicated that she had been doing her desensitization exercises since the time of her tinnitus evaluation, but had misunderstood how "loud" to play the pleasant music and had been playing it "very loudly" for several weeks.

LG called the clinic the following day to indicate that her hearing aids were not working. She was instructed to come into the clinic. She was reinstructed on the features of the hearing aid and the use of the smartphone app. This appeared to resolve the issues.

22.15 Additional Questions for the Reader

1. What other elements, beyond audiology, might the clinician be considering at this point?
2. What other referrals might be necessary?

22.16 Discussion of Additional Questions for the Reader

1. *What other elements, beyond audiology, might the clinician be considering at this point?*
   Many patients with nonspecific dizziness and vague symptoms may have an underlying psychiatric disorder.[3,4] Indeed, in this case, LG had been subjected to a significant traumatic event, and the anxiety could be exacerbating her hearing, tinnitus, and balance symptoms. This case illustrates the value of interprofessional care and dialogue between providers from different disciplines.
2. *What other referrals might be necessary?*
   LG is seeing a behavioral therapist, and embraces a holistic/alternative approach to

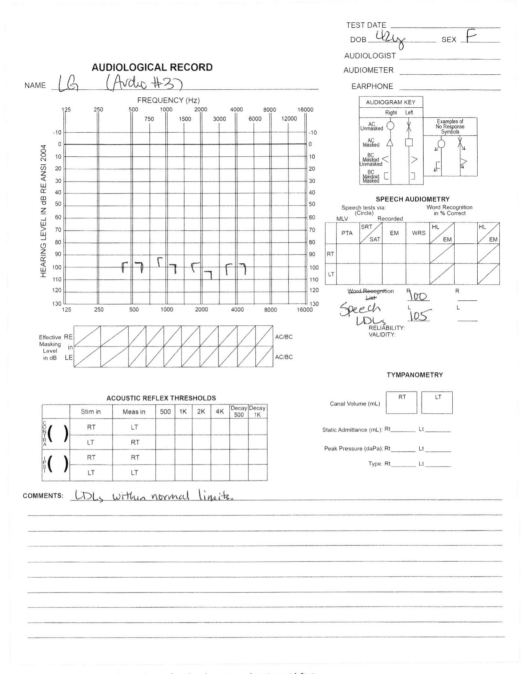

Fig. 22.3 Follow-up loudness discomfort levels prior to hearing aid fitting.

medicine. A referral to a psychiatrist or clinical psychologist should be considered. At this time, we are unaware whether LG has followed through with the recommendation to see other health care providers.

22.17 Self-Efficacy for the Clinician

- Often times there is more to consider about a patient than just tinnitus, hyperacusis, or balance issues. Clinicians are urged to review audiologic scope of practice in order to support their service provision and counseling of patients challenged by multiple conditions.

- Referrals to mental health professionals are often needed for such patients and the provider who establishes viable relationships with providers from other fields should have confidence in their ability to manage a patient's challenges effectively.
- Testing cannot always be completed and decisions sometimes must be made on incomplete diagnoses. The clinician and patient benefit from exclusion of tests that may exacerbate matters for the patient, and the clinician should maintain an up-to-date reading of the literature to support clinical decision-making.

References

[1] Tyler, RS, Pienkowski, M, Roncancio, ER, et al. A review of hyperacusis and future directions: Part I. Definitions and manifestations. American Journal of Audiology. 2014; 23:402–419

[2] Jacobson GP, Newman CW. The development of the Dizziness Handicap Inventory. Arch Otolaryngol Head Neck Surg. 1990 Apr;116(4):424–427. doi: 10.1001/archotol.1990. 01870040046011

[3] Post RE, Dickerson LM. Dizziness: a diagnostic approach. Am Fam Physician. 2010; 82(4):361–368, 369

[4] Brandt T, Huppert D, Strupp M, Dieterich M. Functional dizziness: diagnostic keys and differential diagnosis. J Neurol. 2015; 262(8):1977–1980

Suggested Readings

Bartels H, Middel B, Pedersen SS, Staal MJ, Albers FWJ. The distressed (Type D) personality is independently associated with tinnitus: a case-control study. Psychosomatics. 2010; 51 (1):29–38

Bhatt JM, Bhattacharyya N, Lin HW. Relationships between tinnitus and the prevalence of anxiety and depression. Laryngoscope. 2017; 127(2):466–469

Jüris L, Andersson G, Christian Larsen H, Ekselius L. (2013). Psychiatric comorbidity and personality traits in patients with hyperacusis. Int J Audiol, 52(4Kabat-Zin, J. (2009). Full Catastrophe Living Using the Wisdom of Your Body and Mind to Free Stress, Pain, and Illness, New York, NY: Delta

Udupi VA, Uppunda AK, Mohan KM, Alex J, Mahendra MH. The relationship of perceived severity of tinnitus with depression, anxiety, hearing status, age and gender in individuals with tinnitus. Int Tinnitus J. 2013; 18(1):29–34

23 Tinnitus and Posttraumatic Stress Disorder

Aniruddha K. Deshpande, Colleen A. O'Brien, and Jason H. Thomas

23.1 Clinical History and Description

RM is a 67-year old male seen in the university hearing clinic reporting loud ringing tinnitus in his right ear that began 2 months prior. Shortly before the onset of tinnitus, RM retired as a police detective following an on-the-job injury. He worked in law enforcement for 36 years prior to his retirement. Since retirement, his tinnitus has been constant and extremely bothersome. It fluctuates in intensity and becomes louder at night when he is trying to fall asleep. According to RM, his stress level increased after the onset of his tinnitus, and he reported that the feelings of stress exacerbated tinnitus loudness. He stated that he did not experience tinnitus in the past.

RM denied any noticeable changes in hearing since his retirement. He reported experiencing dizziness on five occasions over the last 2 months. The episodes occurred suddenly and lasted 10 to 20 seconds each. He was unable to identify any specific trigger for these episodes.

23.2 Audiologic Testing

23.2.1 Initial Case History

RM's medical history revealed the following:
- RM takes metformin and dapagliflozin for type 2 diabetes, simvastatin for high cholesterol, and aspirin for occasional headaches; he reported no recent changes in medications.
- He was hospitalized overnight 2 months ago following a superficial gunshot wound to his right shoulder while working as a detective. He received three stitches at the site and was prescribed 10 days of oral antibiotics. He reports the laceration has healed well and there were no further medical complications. He started noticing the tinnitus after the shooting and the retirement – which happened in quick succession.
- RM reported bilateral ear infections—approximately once a year since his youth—and using ear drops prescribed by his physician to treat the infection. The most recent infection occurred 11 months ago. He did not recall the name of the ear drops.

- RM indicated that he has never experienced any vestibular issues in the past. However, his most recent episode of dizziness (2 weeks ago in a grocery store) resulted in a fall. He sustained a bruise to his forehead, but experienced no loss of consciousness. RM reported no serious injuries were sustained from the fall.
- When asked about noise exposure, RM indicated being in close proximity to gunfire throughout his 36-year career in law enforcement. He trained at shooting ranges monthly for at least 25 years of his career. He reported using hearing protection occasionally at the shooting ranges, in the form of disposable earplugs and/or passive supra-aural earmuffs.
- He indicated a family history of presbycusis in his mother and brother.

RM's employment and social history revealed the following:
- RM's involvement in the shooting was his first and only on-the-job injury. A bullet grazed RM's right shoulder and struck his partner's left hand. After being discharged from the hospital, RM decided to retire.
- RM stated that retirement has been difficult since he feels like he is "in shock" after the shooting. He also reported having flashbacks and nightmares related to the event.
- In addition, RM's 90-year-old mother was recently diagnosed with dementia. She lives alone, so he plans to move into her home to serve as her primary caregiver. This situation, in addition to the shooting and retirement, increased his stress level.
- According to RM, his recent episodes of tinnitus and dizziness hindered his daily activities. He reported being hesitant to leave his home in fear that he will have another vestibular episode or worsened tinnitus.

23.2.2 Initial Audiologic Examination (See ▶ Fig. 23.1)

Pure-tone audiometry revealed hearing within normal limits in the low frequencies, sloping precipitously to a severe mixed hearing loss in the mid to high frequencies in the right ear. In the left ear, hearing was within normal limits in the low to

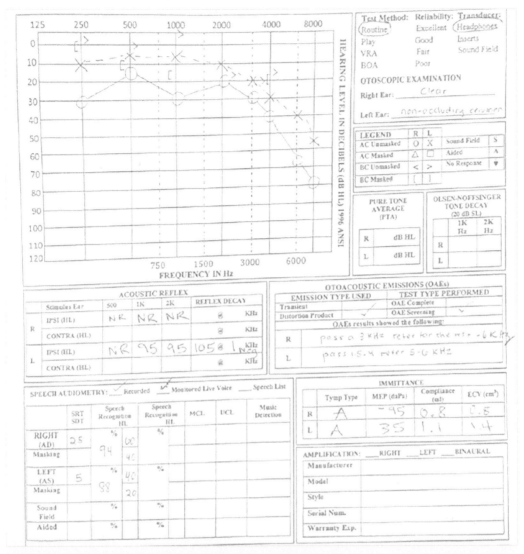

Fig. 23.1 Initial comprehensive audiologic evaluation (CAE) of RM.

mid frequencies, sloping to a moderate mixed hearing loss in the high frequencies, with conductive components at 250, 1,000, and 4,000 Hz. A slight asymmetry was noted, with a greater loss in the right ear. Speech recognition thresholds (SRTs) were 25 dB HL and 5 dB HL in the right and left ears, respectively, which is asymmetrical but consistent with pure-tone findings.[1] In the presence of contralateral masking noise, word recognition scores (WRS) were found to be excellent (94%) in the right ear and good (88%) in the left ear.

Tympanometry revealed ear canal volumes of 0.8 and 1.4 cm³, admittances of 0.8 and 1.1 mL, and middle ear pressures of −95 and 35 daPa in the right and left ears, respectively. Ipsilateral acoustic reflex thresholds (ARTs) were absent at 500, 1,000, and 2,000 Hz in the right ear, which was an unexpected finding based on the pure-tone thresholds. Ipsilateral ARTs in the left ear were absent at 500 Hz and present at 1,000 and 2,000 Hz. Ipsilateral acoustic reflex decay (ARD) test in the left ear was negative and was not tested in the right ear due to the absence of ARTs.

A 6-frequency diagnostic distortion product otoacoustic emission (DPOAE) test was performed bilaterally. The right ear indicated a pass at 3,000 Hz, and referred at 1,500, 2,000, 4,000, 5,000, and 6,000 Hz. In the left ear, DPOAE testing indicated a pass from 1,500 to 4,000 Hz and referred at 5,000 to 6,000 Hz. These findings were consistent with pure-tone results.

The Tinnitus Functional Index (TFI)[2] was administered to determine the functional impact of RM's tinnitus. RM received an overall score of 82 out of 100 points, and a Quality of Life subscale score of 77.5 points. These results suggest that RM's tinnitus had a significant negative impact on his daily life.[3]

23.3 Questions for the Reader

1. What health conditions or lifestyle factors could potentially be contributing to RM's hearing loss and tinnitus?
2. Based on RM's complaints and audiologic results, what additional testing would the reader recommend?

23.4 Discussion of Questions for the Reader

1. *What health conditions or lifestyle factors could potentially be contributing to RM's hearing loss and tinnitus?*

   RM has a history of long-standing occupational noise exposure, which may have contributed to his current high-frequency hearing loss, absent DPOAEs, and absent ARTs. Positioning firearms on the right side at shooting ranges (due to his right handedness) may explain the greater degree of hearing loss in his right ear. RM also reported a long history of ear infections that may have contributed to his air-bone gaps and acoustic reflex findings.

   It is noteworthy that RM reported developing tinnitus, dizziness, stress, anxiety, flashbacks, and nightmares immediately following his involvement in a shooting and subsequent retirement. Psychological factors may have exacerbated some of his symptoms, as several of his complaints were consistent with posttraumatic stress disorder (PTSD). PTSD is a condition characterized by many symptoms of hyperarousal and distress that may develop after an individual experiences a life-threatening event. Symptoms such as anxiety and re-experiencing the trauma (i.e., flashbacks) may last for several months to years, and hinder daily function.[4] Recent investigations reported a relationship between PTSD and development of tinnitus memories.[5] Tinnitus may serve as a stimulus related to the initial distressing event, ultimately producing or amplifying anxiety, stress, and fear related to the tinnitus perception.[6] RM's mother's recent dementia diagnosis and associated lifestyle changes may also be additional exacerbating stressors.

2. *Based on RM's complaints and audiologic results, what additional testing would the reader recommend?*

   Physician referral: It is pertinent for RM to follow up with his physician or an ear-nose-throat specialist (ENT) to investigate atypical findings of asymmetry of hearing thresholds and presence of unilateral tinnitus. RM was seen by his ENT shortly after his audiologic evaluation. The ENT's physical examination did not reveal any noteworthy findings, and the ENT did not suspect that RM's tinnitus and dizziness were caused by any of his medications.

   Neuroimaging: Neuroimaging testing would be valuable in determining if there is an anatomical cause for his asymmetrical hearing thresholds and unilateral tinnitus. RM was referred for imaging by his ENT to rule out any physical causes of his symptoms. Magnetic resonance imaging (MRI) scanning of RM's inner ears and surrounding structures was unremarkable bilaterally, with no significant anatomical anomalies noted. RM's ENT suspects that mixed components are related to a long-term history of bilateral otitis media. The ENT provided medical clearance for amplification and made a referral for a psychological evaluation to determine the involvement of past trauma and poor stress management.

   Vestibular testing: RM was referred by his ENT for a vestibular assessment in light of recent episodes of dizziness. He was seen in the university clinic for videonystagmography (VNG), positional, and caloric testing. No vestibular symptoms were noted at the time of testing. All results of VNG, Dix Hallpike maneuver, and caloric testing were within normal limits. Slight nystagmus was noted during gaze testing. This was determined to be an insignificant finding.

   Psychiatrist referral: It is clear that RM experienced physical and psychological trauma related to being shot by a suspect while working as a police detective. A referral to a psychiatrist or other professional trained in managing PTSD would be critical because the skills required to manage PTSD symptoms fall outside the scope of an audiologist. RM was referred to a psychiatrist by his ENT.

23.5 Final Diagnosis and Recommended Treatment

RM was determined to have mixed hearing loss, likely due to noise exposure and long-term bilateral otitis media. Bilateral amplification and tinnitus programs were recommended after RM was given medical clearance for amplification by his ENT. He was given bilateral Widex Evoke 440 receiver-in-the canal (RIC) combination instruments with the Widex Zen Therapy tinnitus program. The Widex Zen Therapy intake questionnaire revealed that RM falls within Level 4 (severe negative reaction to tinnitus). He was given four Zen programs: Zen Lavender, Zen noise, and two variations of Zen Aqua. He was also counseled on use of the Widex Zen mobile application to adjust his tinnitus management programs throughout the day.

RM indicated that he will likely continue to participate in shooting ranges as a leisure activity. Over-the-counter hearing protection solutions and custom devices were discussed. Due to his current and prior history of noise exposure, as well as concerns about worsening tinnitus, RM decided to obtain custom-molded earplugs with two filter options.

After completing a psychological evaluation, RM was diagnosed with PTSD related to his shooting involvement several months prior. His psychiatrist determined that his flashbacks and nightmares were likely capable of exacerbating his newly developed tinnitus and vestibular issues. It was also revealed that RM was feeling a great deal of guilt that his partner sustained more serious injuries than his. Additional stressors involving his mother's recent dementia diagnosis were also discussed. RM and his psychiatrist decided to employ cognitive behavioral therapy (CBT) to help RM manage his reaction to the prior trauma. CBT is a psychological treatment that focuses on altering adverse thoughts, reactions, and actions based on past traumas, and learning to implement more constructive and positive thought processes.[7] CBT is also effective in managing reactions to tinnitus.[6]

Finally, RM was asked to return for annual audiologic evaluations to monitor thresholds.

23.6 Outcomes

23.6.1 Hearing Aid Outcomes

At his 1-month follow-up appointment, RM reported high satisfaction with his Widex hearing aids and Zen programs. Data logging revealed an average of 14 hours of daily use. He indicated that he generally uses the first Zen Aqua program, and his tinnitus has become much less noticeable. Aided soundfield testing assessed using AzBio sentences[8] in quiet revealed a score of 94%, compared to 76% unaided, suggesting good aided benefit from his Widex devices.

23.6.2 Cognitive Behavioral Therapy Outcomes

RM and his psychiatrist met weekly for 60-minute sessions, during which they utilized psychological counseling tools to minimize RM's adverse reactions to his flashbacks, guilt, and tinnitus. After 20 weeks of CBT sessions, RM reported significant reduction in anxiety and negative thoughts related to his shooting. RM shared that when he now has a "bad day," he has learned to adjust his automatic and exaggerated negative beliefs into more accurate and constructive thoughts. He believes that this technique has helped him to manage his tinnitus as well. He still experiences tinnitus in his right ear while trying to fall asleep, but he reported that the tinnitus is now significantly less bothersome than it had been in the past.

23.6.3 Audiologic Follow-Up

RM was then seen 6 months after his initial appointment for a follow-up audiologic re-evaluation to monitor his hearing thresholds (see ▶ Fig. 23.2). His medication list remained unchanged. RM denied any changes in hearing and reported a reduction in annoyance caused by his tinnitus. He also experienced only one additional episode of lightheadedness since his VNG testing, which he believes was caused by dehydration.

Pure-tone audiologic testing revealed a slight improvement in hearing thresholds in the low frequencies in the right ear from the previous evaluation, likely due to the resolution of conductive components. An asymmetrical hearing loss remained, particularly in the high frequencies, with the right ear continuing to be poorer than the left ear. RM also had an opaque right tympanic membrane, and tympanometry revealed high compliance in the right ear, suggestive of excessive tympanic membrane mobility in the right ear. In addition, ARTs were absent at all tested frequencies bilaterally.

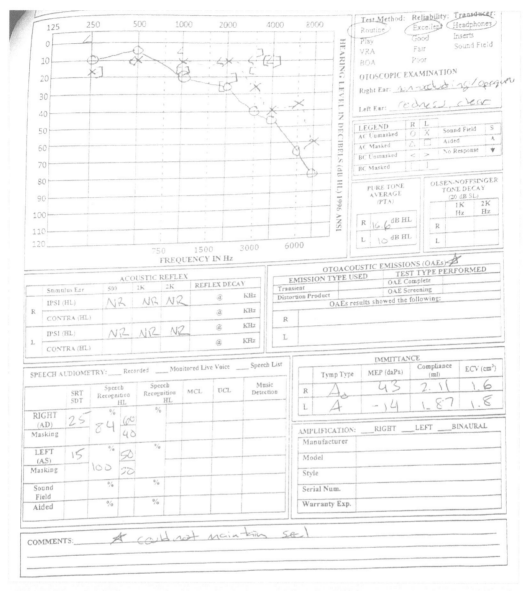

Fig. 23.2 Six-month follow-up comprehensive audiologic evaluation (CAE) for RM.

The TFI was readministered at RM's 6-month follow-up appointment. Overall score decreased from 82 points at baseline to 60.4 points out of 100, and the Quality of Life subscale decreased from 77.5 to 57.5 points. These findings indicate that the negative impacts of RM's tinnitus were minimized, suggesting that he learned to better cope with the condition compared to baseline.

23.7 Key Points

- Obtaining a thorough and accurate case history is critical when assessing a patient for newly developed tinnitus.
- Tinnitus can be exacerbated by stressful situations related to past trauma.
- Audiologists must be aware of when a case falls outside of their scope, and warrants

referral to another provider, including ENT and psychiatry.

- CBT is a highly effective means of managing tinnitus, especially when present in conjunction with other mental health conditions.

References

[1] Katz J, Chasin M, English KM, Hood LJ, Tillery KL. Handbook of clinical audiology. Philadelphia, PA: Wolters Kluwer; 2015

[2] Meikle, MB, Henry, JA, Griest, SE, et al. The tinnitus functional index: development of a new clinical measure for chronic, intrusive tinnitus. *Ear and hearing.* 2012;33(2): 153–176

[3] Henry, JA, Griest, S, Thielman, E, et al. Tinnitus functional index: development, validation, outcomes research, and clinical application. Hearing Research. 2016;334:58–64

[4] Mayo Clinic. Post-traumatic stress disorder (PTSD). Mayo Clinic; 2018. Retrieved from https://www.mayoclinic.org/ diseases-conditions/post-traumatic-stress-disorder/ symptoms-causes/syc-20355967

[5] Moring JC, Peterson AL, Kanzler KE. Tinnitus, traumatic brain injury, and posttraumatic stress disorder in the military. Int J Behav Med. 2018; 25(3):312–321

[6] Cima RF, Andersson G, Schmidt CJ, Henry JA. Cognitive-behavioral treatments for tinnitus: a review of the literature. J Am Acad Audiol. 2014; 25(1):29–61

[7] Jun HJ, Park MK. Cognitive behavioral therapy for tinnitus: evidence and efficacy. Korean J Audiol. 2013; 17 (3):101–104

[8] Spahr AJ, Dorman MF, Litvak LM, et al. Development and validation of the AzBio sentence lists. Ear Hear. 2012; 33(1): 112–117

Suggested Reading

Dawes P, Cruickshanks KJ, Marsden A, Moore DR, Munro KJ. Relationship between diet, tinnitus, and hearing difficulties. Ear Hear. 2020; 41(2):289–299

Section B: Psychological Correlates

II: Disorders of Sound Tolerance

24 Poor Outcome in Misophonia Intervention despite Evidence-Based Intervention Strategies

Michael Hoffman, Jenna M. Pellicori, and Tammy Riegner

24.1 Clinical History and Description

A 14-year-old female and her family initially sought services for sound intolerance through occupational therapy due to sensory concerns. The family's objective was to obtain strategies to decrease auditory sensitivity, which was associated with the patient's tactile defensiveness, reports of frequent and debilitating anxiety, and sensory overload. An occupational therapist administered the Sensory Profile 2 Child Assessment, and the patient was referred to audiology due to concerns for possible hyperacusis with notable auditory and oral aversions.

At the audiology consultation appointment, the family reported hypersensitivity to loud noises and typically occurring environmental sounds (e.g., church music, chewing noises during school lunch, breathing sounds) as well as feelings of being overwhelmed in crowded environments such as the mall, hallways, and school cafeteria. In addition, the patient reported that the sound of clicking pens, feet shuffling, and oral movements were notably bothersome. In particular, sounds of chewing, sniffling, or pen/pencil tapping caused her to feel "frustrated, upset, angry" and experience a great deal of "anxiety." According to the mother, these episodes occurred multiple times daily, both at home and school.

The patient's medical and birth history were remarkable—she was born prematurely at 30 weeks gestation with a birth weight of < 3 pounds; she required admission to the neonatal intensive care unit (NICU) for approximately 1½ months. The patient passed her newborn hearing screen at birth in both ears per parent report. There was no family history of childhood hearing loss reported; however, the patient's mother noted similar auditory behaviors in the maternal grandmother, suggesting a possible family history or inheritance. The patient's medical history included a previous diagnosis by her primary care physician, of Sensory Processing Disorder (SPD) and Generalized Anxiety Disorder (GAD).

Based upon case history reports and the report of symptoms gathered during the audiology appointment, annoyance hyperacusis, or misophonia, was suspected. The patient had not yet met with a psychologist to address these concerns but such a consultation was discussed with the family.

24.2 Audiological Testing

Otoscopy revealed nonoccluding cerumen in both ears with intact tympanic membranes. Impedance measures were performed bilaterally and revealed normal middle ear system compliance and pressure, consistent with normal middle ear function. Ipsilateral and contralateral middle ear muscle reflex testing was tolerated, and reflexes were present from 500 to 4,000 Hz in both ears in all ipsilateral and left contralateral conditions. Right contralateral reflexes were absent at all four frequencies at a 100 dB HL presentation level. The ipsilateral findings indicate synchrony throughout the middle ear acoustic reflex arc and contraindicate auditory neuropathy spectrum disorder (ANSD). Distortion product otoacoustic emissions (DPOAE) were evaluated from 2,000 to 6,000 Hz and were present bilaterally, supporting the likelihood of normal cochlear outer hair cell function for the frequency range evaluated. It should be noted that the patient did not demonstrate any tactile or sensory aversions during the aforementioned objective measures.

Conventional audiometric testing was conducted using behavioral means for assessment. Speech recognition thresholds (SRTs) using monitored live voice and spondee words were estimated at 5 dB HL for both ears. A Word Recognition Score (WRS) with a presentation level of 40 dB SL (re: SRT) was obtained at 100% in quiet bilaterally and 96% in noise (+ 5 dB signal-to-noise ratio (SNR) in the ipsilateral channel) for both ears. The patient's responses to pulsed pure tones fell within the normal range of hearing from 250 to 8,000 Hz, at octave and interoctave (1.5, 3, and 6 kHz) frequencies bilaterally. Ultra/extended high frequencies were also evaluated and revealed thresholds ranging from −20 dBSPL to 10 dBSPL from 9,000 to 20,000 Hz, within, or slightly better than, accepted values at those frequencies. The SRT and pure-tone averages were in agreement bilaterally, indicating good test reliability and normal hearing sensitivity.

The uncomfortable loudness levels (UCLs), the level or intensity of a sound at which a patient reports sound to be uncomfortably loud, were obtained from 500 to 4,000 Hz for both ears. The loudness discomfort levels fell within a clinically acceptable range (≥ 90 dB HL); the patient's dynamic range was clearly not the source of her sound intolerance, which along with her report and history eliminates the likelihood of loudness hyperacusis.

24.3 Additional Audiological Testing

The patient returned for central auditory system assessment intended to identify involvement within the central auditory nervous system (CANS). Cortical (or late) auditory evoked potentials (CAEP) were obtained while the patient was awake and in a state of calm repose while watching a silenced video screen. The CAEP test is an objective measure of the neuromaturation of the higher auditory pathway and assesses ability to detect speech stimuli in quiet and varying noise conditions. A four-electrode, dual-channel montage was used with ER-3A insert earphones to present a /da/ stimulus in quiet, ipsilateral noise, and binaural noise paradigms. Noise conditions had a + 5 signal-to-noise ratio (SNR) with an 80 dBSPL stimulus and 75 dBSPL noise. Findings showed absent responses of the P1/N1 and P2/N2 bilaterally in all three test conditions. This is an indication that the auditory cortex is not efficiently detecting and responding to incoming speech information in quiet and noise conditions.

In addition, suppression of transient-evoked otoacoustic emissions (TEOAEs) was performed while the patient was awake and attending to a quiet visual activity. OAE suppression assesses a reflexive system believed to help in the processing of speech sounds in the presence of background noise, the Medial Olivo-Cochlear System (MOCS). ER-100 OAE probes were used to present a 65 dBSPL click to each ear in the presence of ipsilateral noise (+ 5 dBSNR). With ipsilateral noise present, while there was a normal amount of suppression occurring in both ears, in the left ear, a reduced OAE suppression value was noted in comparison to the right ear. Some caution in interpretation should be taken, given that fewer measures were taken in the left ear. The difference in suppression between ears was 7.21 dB, which was well outside normative values (less than 2 dB) for asymmetry

in this condition. This suggests that the right ear may be more effective at reducing the effects of background noise in more challenging listening situations. While the importance of this difference is not known at this time, other patients with misophonia at our clinic have shown similar asymmetry when they have had this testing. Further research is warranted, given some of these initial indications, and while there is no published data to support these claims, the authors currently are conducting research in this area.

The Misophonia Assessment Questionnaire[1] was completed to better ascertain the patient's perceived degree of impairment. A total score of 25 was obtained, which indicates a subjective severity rating of "moderate" range.

Based on these findings, a case can be made that further evaluation of the CANS as well as the MOCS may prove beneficial in identifying multiple physiological sources in central pathways for these auditory symptoms. Identifying areas of pathophysiology may help professionals on the multidisciplinary team more effectively manage the perceptually overwhelming symptoms.

24.4 Questions for the Reader

1. What are the typical audiologic findings in patients with annoyance hyperacusis/misophonia?
2. Could heightened sensitivity to ultra/extended high frequencies be exacerbating the underlying sensitivity to certain sounds?
3. The patient was initially referred to audiology due to concerns for annoyance hyperacusis and concerns for sound intolerance. What is the difference in symptoms between loudness hyperacusis and annoyance hyperacusis (misophonia)? Can the two conditions be comorbid or correlated?
4. How can an integrated, multidisciplinary care model be used to provide comprehensive services to these patients? What role can disciplines such as psychology play when providing treatment?

24.5 Discussion of Questions for the Reader

1. *What are the typical audiologic findings in patients with annoyance hyperacusis/misophonia?*
   Patients with misophonia present with varying

hearing acuity; however, the literature suggests that the majority of patients diagnosed with misophonia will have normal peripheral hearing sensitivity at the time of their initial diagnosis. A study by Schroder et al[2] provided 20 patients with misophonia a comprehensive hearing assessment using pure tones, speech, and loudness discomfort levels and reported no peripheral deficits among the participants. Although the exact physiological and psychological mechanisms of misophonia are not yet fully understood, research suggests that the heightened state of the limbic and autonomic nervous system may be the potential origin for the abnormal adverse reaction to certain every day auditory stimuli, due to the excitation of certain brain pathways, and is likely not the result of an abnormality in the peripheral auditory system.[3]

2. *Could heightened sensitivity to ultra/extended high frequencies be exacerbating the underlying sensitivity to certain sounds?*
More research is required in this area before any definitive conclusions can be drawn. Clinical audiologists do not typically test above 8,000 Hz in routine clinical practice; however, people are born with a range of hearing from 20 to 20,000 Hz and the current indication is that people often begin to lose the ultra/extended high frequencies early in life. Although the average age of decline is not well established, common thought is that this likely begins in later adolescence. Normative data for pediatric ultra/extended high-frequency evaluation should be researched before any definitive conclusions can be drawn from this data.

3. *The patient was initially referred to an audiologist due to concerns for hyperacusis. What is the difference between hyperacusis and misophonia? Can the two conditions be comorbid or correlated?*
The terms "misophonia" and "hyperacusis" are often confused in the health care community because both terms fall under the realm of "decreased sound tolerance disorders." Despite this generalized similarity, it is reasonable to consider misophonia as a type of hyperacusis, specifically "annoyance hyperacusis" as suggested by Tyler et al.[4]
Misophonia, or annoyance hyperacusis, refers to an adverse response to, in most cases, soft-repetitive pattern-based sounds (e.g., sniffling, chewing, breathing, and pen-clicking). A patient

with misophonia may react differently to stimuli depending on the situation and source of the sound but adverse reactions are extremely intense, often to the point of rage and/or extreme anxiety, similar to the response that would be expected by hearing a sound of great, and usually negative value; the problem is that the response to such sounds is disproportionate to the sounds' value. These patients also commonly react to visual triggers as well. This is thought to result from enhanced functional connections between the auditory, limbic, and autonomic nervous system that can be triggered by specific sounds for some people.[5,6]

Loudness hyperacusis, on the other hand, is a collapsed dynamic range and intolerance to normal environmental sounds of moderate-to-high intensity[5]; most professionals consider the term "hyperacusis" to refer in a limited fashion to the experience of excessive loudness to sound levels that do not bother other people, and that do not damage the auditory mechanism. These patients experience reduced UCL responses in addition to subjective complaints of sound intolerance. Hyperacusis often depends on the physical characteristics of the sound, and the patient will often respond consistently to the same sound in all situations.[5]

4. *How can an integrated, multidisciplinary care model be used to provide comprehensive services to these patients? What role can disciplines such as psychology play when providing treatment?*
Many patients with sound sensitivities experience comorbid psychological diagnoses, including anxiety, depression, and adjustment disorder. The interaction between sound sensitivities and mental health challenges can exacerbate symptoms, contribute to aversions and withdrawal, and reduce the patient's quality of life. Providing audiological treatment in conjunction with psychological services facilitates well-rounded care, including teaching the patient coping strategies when they are experiencing difficulties related to sound sensitivities or self-regulation. Research has shown cognitive behavioral therapy (CBT) intervention, perhaps including desensitization strategies, to be particularly beneficial for patients diagnosed with decreased sound tolerance disorders.

24.6 Final Diagnosis and Recommended Treatment

The patient was referred to psychology for consultation and CBT, at which point a diagnosis of misophonia was provided. CBT, in this application, employed teaching strategies to improve coping with sound sensitivities, including thought restructuring, problem-solving, mindfulness, and self-advocacy. Treatment also involved components to Acceptance and Commitment Therapy, which centered on helping the patient engage in meaningful life activities while not allowing the misophonia to inhibit their daily functioning. The patient also received a brief course of biofeedback training. This involved teaching diaphragmatic breathing intended to support parasympathetic nervous system activity when the patient experienced physiological arousal (e.g., increased heart rate and body temperature) due to the triggering sounds.

In addition to psychological intervention, the audiology department recommended the implementation of a trial with sound therapy using ear-level sound generator devices. Sound therapy was centered on using broadband and environmental sounds (e.g., ocean waves, rain, and thunder), to reduce the patient's ability to detect and react to softer, more bothersome sounds. The goal was to incorporate sound therapy to help mask the trigger sounds, thereby reducing the response to the aversive stimuli while introducing more pleasant auditory experiences in their place.

The use of sound putatively supports behavioral therapy intervention that supports coping mechanisms, as the patient has the ability to increase the masker, or background stimulus, thereby decreasing the degree to which the triggering sound stands out against the acoustic background. The patient is encouraged to incorporate and practice breathing exercises and management techniques, in order to reduce arousal and the sense of aversion prior to re-entering the auditory environment. Sound therapy should preserve speech recognition as it reduces or eliminates the response to the trigger sound. Ideally, patients would not have to physically remove or isolate themselves from the environment, and would feel an improved sense of control over their surroundings.

24.7 Outcome

Despite the introduction and implementation of numerous techniques shown to be effective in the literature, including CBT, Acceptance and Commitment Therapy, biofeedback training, and the implementation of sound therapy, the patient frequently reported that these strategies had limited benefit. The patient and her family decided to return the ear-level sound generator devices to the manufacturer, as she did not demonstrate any meaningful improvement or benefit with these devices. She continues to be seen through the behavioral health department for psychological services. The family is still seeking alternative treatment and management plans in hopes of improved outcomes for their child.

References

[1] Johnson M, Dozier T. Misophonia Assessment Questionnaire (MAQ). July 2013. Retrieved from http://csd.wp.uncg.edu/wp-content/uploads/sites/6/2014/03/MAQ.pdf

[2] Schröder A, Vulink N, Denys D. Misophonia: diagnostic criteria for a new psychiatric disorder. PLoS One. 2013; 8(1): e54706

[3] Møller, AR. "Misophonia, phonophobia, and "exploding head" syndrome." Textbook of Tinnitus. Springer, New York, NY, 2011. 25–27

[4] Tyler RS, Pienkowski M, Roncancio ER, et al. A review of hyperacusis and future directions: part I. Definitions and manifestations. Am J Audiol. 2014; 23(4):402–419

[5] Jastreboff PJ, Jastreboff MM. Treatment for decreased sound tolerance (hyperacusis and misophonia). Semin Hear. 2014; 35(2):105–120

[6] Kumar S, Tansley-Hancock O, Sedley W, et al. The brain basis for misophonia. Curr Biol. 2017; 27(4):527–533

Suggested Readings

Goldstein B, Shulman A. Tinnitus—Hyperacusis and the loudness discomfort level test: a preliminary report. Int Tinnitus J. 1996; 2:83–89

Schröder A, van Diepen R, Mazaheri A, et al. Diminished n1 auditory evoked potentials to oddball stimuli in misophonia patients. Front Behav Neurosci. 2014; 8(123):123

25 LM ("Lisa"): Coping Skills Development for Misophonia

Jennifer Jo Brout

25.1 Clinical History and Description

LM is a 16-year-old girl, in the eleventh grade referred for coping skills training by her audiologist. LM's parents reported that Lisa reached all developmental milestones within normal limits, her health history unremarkable, and her academic history excellent. Currently, Lisa attends her local public high school. She is in honors classes and has a grade average of A-. She has always been highly social. She has a 19-year-old sister who attends college and lives out of the house during most of the school year. Lisa is athletic and is on her local and travel soccer and basketball teams.

Mr. and Mrs. M expressed concerned that since Lisa was approximately 13 to 14 years old, she was overly sensitive to certain sounds. Neither Mr. nor Mrs. M was certain when the problem started. However, they each recalled their otherwise "well-adjusted and happy teenager breaking down during a family dinner." When asked to describe this, Lisa's mother explained that during a typical family dinner, seemingly "out of nowhere" Lisa put her head down at the table and began to cry. When her parents queried, Lisa would not answer and ran into her bedroom. After this incident, Lisa refused to eat with her family again. The M's assumed that their daughter was experiencing "typical teenage behavior" (i.e., mood swings and preference to spend time with peers over family). Therefore, the M's decided to allow their daughter the "space" they felt she needed and did not force her to eat dinner with them or to explain why.

After 3 months, the Ms' became much more concerned, as they felt their daughter had become more isolated from friends as well as family. At this point, Lisa's parents insisted that she see a psychiatrist for at least one visit, even though Lisa was highly resistant to this idea. The psychiatrist suggested to the Ms' that their daughter may have an obsessive compulsive and related disorder (OCD). The psychiatrist pointed out that, given Lisa's high grades and membership on numerous athletic teams, LM seemed to have a "perfectionistic personality." The psychiatrist also stated that Lisa "ruminates on things...especially sounds." Lastly, the psychiatrist added that during the session, Lisa mentioned a disorder that she thought she may have called "misophonia" that she had read about on the Internet. The psychiatrist stated that while he had heard about this disorder, he did not "believe in it." He suggested that the M's follow up with cognitive behavioral therapy (CBT) for OCD and possibly medication if Lisa did not improve.

The M's followed the direction of the psychiatrist, and Lisa saw a psychologist for CBT. However, after three sessions of CBT, Lisa refused to attend. The last time that the M's tried to convince Lisa to leave for therapy, Lisa became very angry. According to Mr. and Mrs. M, they had never seen Lisa so angry. Reportedly, she locked herself in her room and refused to come out. The next morning, Lisa would not go to school. Her parents did not know what to do. They called Lisa's CBT therapist, Dr. W, for guidance. Dr. W explained that he was not sure that the OCD diagnosis was correct. He had heard of misophonia and thought Lisa should be assessed for this. He gave the M's the name of a local audiologist who he was reasonably sure knew about misophonia.

25.2 Audiology Report

According to the audiology report, pure-tone testing revealed that hearing was within normal limits bilaterally. Word recognition in quiet was excellent and tympanograms indicated normal middle ear function. Otoacoustic emissions were present from 0.750 to 10 kHz bilaterally, suggesting normal outer hair cell function for these frequencies. LM's responses to questions regarding sound and her tolerance of signals in excess of 90 dB HL contraindicated presence of loudness hyperacusis. LM did not describe any symptoms of tinnitus. The audiologist fitted LM with ear-level sound generators and explained how to use them. Specifically, LM was instructed to wear the sound generators as frequently as possible. The sound generators produced broad brand white noise, in order to interfere with the trigger sounds' negative effects, as they allowed for other sounds to be heard.

25.3 Questions for the Reader

1. What do you think accounted for the sudden change in Lisa's behavior at home?
2. Why is CBT alone not an appropriate treatment for misophonia?
3. What accounts for the confusion between OCD and misophonia?
4. Why is it also important to distinguish hyperacusis from hyperacusis (misophonia)? Note: Hyperacusis is a disorder in which sounds are perceived louder than subjectively measured.
5. What course of action should be considered if the individual feels the ear-level sound generators are uncomfortable?

25.4 Discussion of Questions for the Reader

1. *What do you think accounted for the sudden change in Lisa's behavior at home?*
   There are a number of possibilities to account for Lisa's sudden behavioral change. Because we do not know her age at onset nor when hyperacusis, or misophonia first manifested, her behavior may reflect the first time she experienced misophonia.[1,2] More likely, it is possible that she was aware of her reactivity to specific auditory stimuli and better able to contain her response until the family dinner incident. In addition, other life stressors (e.g., hormonal changes, social issues related to adolescence, and school pressure) may have made her more vulnerable to reactivity.

2. *Why is CBT alone not an appropriate treatment for misophonia?*
   CBT is helpful. However, CBT on its own may not adequately address the range of symptoms associated with misophonia.[1,2] Elements of CBT that are often helpful include reframing the trigger (i.e., separating trigger sounds from people). In addition, CBT can be combined with auditory devices (such as sound generators), auditory therapy (using sound generators to habituate to sounds),[3] and occupational therapy (in order to address other sensory issues [if present] as well as teaching self-regulation).[4,5] Psychoeducation is also important, as it facilitates combining these other therapies into practical coping skills. Most important, research has demonstrated that exposure therapy (a form of CBT) may be detrimental to those with misophonia.[6]

3. *What accounts for the confusion between OCD and misophonia?*
   Misophonia is often mistaken for OCD because it appears that the individual is "obsessing on sounds and/or ruminating on sounds." However, while the two disorders can be comorbid, they are distinct from one another.[8,10] In general OCD involves internal stimuli (thoughts), whereas a misophonic reactivity is activated by external stimuli (sounds) that are processed in a manner consistent with a signal of importance and substantial negative value. Kumar et al[11] compared functional connectivity in auditory and emotional areas of the brain and reported sounds that triggered misophonic responses produced substantial activity in emotional centers that far exceeded the activity in control participants without sound aversions. Their findings demonstrated that patients with specific sound aversions displayed brain activity commensurate with their assigning value to sounds (such as silverware clattering) that unaffected individuals did not. The powerful responses displayed by such individuals were limited to trigger sounds and were not observed when the patients heard annoying sounds (such as children crying) or neutral sounds (such as running water). Recent reserearch by Kumar et al discovered that the primary motor cortex is involved in misophonia. Specifically when a person with misophonia sees another person chewing (for example) they have something akin to a premonitary urge to mimic the action. Kumer et al's findings are supported by MRI scans showing a higher number of mirror neurons around the oral/nasal areas of the misophonic. This research is certainly the beginning of a better understanding to the underlying neurological mechanisms of misophonia.[9]

4. *Why is it also important to distinguish hyperacusis from hyperacusis (misophonia)? Note: Hyperacusis is a disorder in which sounds are perceived louder than subjectively measured.*
   It is important to distinguish these types of sound intolerance because these two disorders are often confused with one another. Further, interventions including coping skills development differ for each, as well as for rarer cases in which an individual has both.[12] For example, individuals with misophonia (without loudness intolerance) are often able to use maskers to reduce some

of the discomfort produced by the pattern-based and repetitive quieter sounds that bother them when in a loud environment. Some, but not all, find for example that they can eat dinner with family and friends in loud restaurants, whereas such strategies might not be well-tolerated by a patient with loudness hyperacusis.

5. *What course of action should be considered if the individual feels the ear-level sound generators are uncomfortable?*

   It is very important that the patient work with an audiologist and that the audiologist lets the patient know that if at any time the ear-level sound generators are uncomfortable, the device output can be reduced. Similarly, it is important that psychologists and counselors communicate with their patients' audiologists if an individual is experiencing discomfort with sound-generating devices so that other choices may be explored (e.g., headphones, etc.).

25.5 Diagnosis and Treatment Plan (Coping Skills Development)

25.5.1 General Description

Coping skills development for individuals with annoyance hyperacusis, or misophonia, should be individually based and include a combination of the following:

1. Psychoeducation.
2. Physiological regulation skills.
3. Cognitive reframing.
4. Empathic understanding.
5. Practically based solutions.

25.6 Specific Case Intervention Discussion and Outcome

I initially met with LM and her parents for an hour, in order to obtain her developmental, health, and academic history. LM's parents agreed to leave the room so that I could establish a rapport with LM in order to assess how misophonia was influencing various areas of her life, as well as to set intervention goals. LM began crying when her parents left the room, explaining that she felt that she was a terrible disappointment to her parents, and that she felt that she was "cursed" by misophonia. When queried, she explained that she had been

reading on the Internet and was terrified that her "triggers were spreading" and that she would eventually end up isolated, both tormented by others and hateful of them. She said she was so angry when people chewed, sniffled, or tapped on a keyboard that she felt she had become a monster. She described either crying when triggered and/or feeling as though she had to "get away."

I began by debunking the misinformation Lisa had garnered on the Internet and assured her that she was in fact doing very well, and that I was certain that, with coping skills on board, she would be able to manage her life despite misophonia. During this session, psychoeducation was used in order to help Lisa understand the mechanisms underlying the misophonia experience. Psychoeducation is often the first step in coping skills development (P. Jastreboff, personal communication, July 24, 2018). I explained to Lisa that misophonia is not a psychiatric or personality disorder. It is an auditory and neurologically based disorder. Here is a simple explanation:

In misophonia, sounds are misinterpreted as toxic or harmful. In response, the body goes into the fight/flight response. This happens within milliseconds and is outside conscious awareness or control. When the fight/flight response is triggered, the affected individual may feel an overwhelming need to either "flee" or "fight" the perceived triggering source. Cognitions and emotions, of course, are involved. However, the feelings begin with an automatic process that is similar to reactions associated with survival.[12]

Lisa stated that she was so relieved to understand what was happening to her, that it was neurologically based and that she "wasn't crazy" or "a terrible person." She said that thinking of the fight/flight response made so much sense to her. When triggered she always wants to leave (flee) and if she could not leave, she felt overwhelmed by anger (which she now recognized as an "emotion word" related to "fight").

At the end of the session, Lisa agreed to tell her parents how she was feeling. Her parents were highly empathic and told her that they were there to help her in whatever way she needed. Regarding meal time, I suggested that Lisa continue to eat separately until coping skills were more developed. The family agreed. We briefly discussed her other triggers, and I suggested that the family not modify their behavior extensively (but be mindful of Lisa's physiological and emotional reactions).

We agreed that I would see Lisa for 10 sessions. Over the 10 sessions, we worked on the following:

1. **Separating sounds from the people who make them**

   Lisa often referred to her father, and a specific teacher, as her triggers. I explained that it was important to refer to the sounds, and not the specific people, as triggers. Lisa asked me why her father's chewing was worse than her mother's chewing. She said that she adored her father and that this did not make sense to her. I explained that research has not yet delineated why the sounds produced by some people would be worse than others. There could be acoustical or memory processes of which we are not yet aware that combine to make some people more difficult to tolerate than others. However, there is no correlation between how one feels about someone and the extent to which that person's sounds are bothersome. Often, in fact, it is the people who we love most that bother us the most. I assured her that this does not have to impair a relationship.

2. **Alternative family activities**

   Lisa asked me how she could possibly make her relationship with her father better when she cannot "even sit with him at dinner." We went over numerous activities that she and her father could do together that did not involve eating and in which other trigger sounds would be minimized. Often when people are outdoors and/or in motion, the senses are processed differently.[13,14] Lisa lit up when I said that, as she realized that she does much better when she is outside and when she is moving. Lisa said that she was going to talk to her father, and they made a list of activities that they could do together.

3. **General arousal level**

   Since we know that the fight/flight response is activated by sound,[15] it is always helpful to find activities that help an individual with misophonia stay at a lower arousal level. Since Lisa loved athletics, I was able to use this to help her. Again, using psychoeducation I explained that when the sympathetic nervous system is aroused, the parasympathetic system engages so that the individual reaches homeostasis again. From the field of occupational therapy, we know that exercises that involve the proprioceptive system help bring in the parasympathetic response. Lisa and I went

through activities that she could do regularly in order to keep sympathetic arousal in check, as well as exercises she could do "in the moment" when triggered.

- Weight lifting (Lisa would keep hand weights in her room).
- 4 Square breathing.
- Hand gripper.

   As coping skills treatment continued, Lisa began to understand that she had more control over her physiological response than she had previously believed. She also became very clear that those she loved were not her "triggers" but that "certain sounds were." While she still found it difficult to eat with her family, she felt much more in control of her life in general. She also felt less guilty about her effect on family meals, and about times in which she had to excuse herself and either retreat to her room, utilize her headphones, and/or leave for a "break" until she felt physiologically calm. Helping an individual with misophonia rewrite their narrative by providing an accurate lexicon and strategies to improve self-talk is a very important step.

4. **Anticipatory anxiety**

   As Lisa gained more control, her anticipatory anxiety was also reduced. This is very important and is a reciprocal and integrative process. When one feels out of control, anxiety peaks. When anxiety spikes, arousal level is higher. When arousal level is higher, reactivity to sounds will likely increase.

   While our work together progressed, Lisa came in one day quite upset (around the seventh session). She noticed that now just seeing a person chewing triggered her. It did not matter if she heard the sound or not.

5. **Visual stimuli**

   Triggering stimuli may unfortunately become associated with auditory and visual inputs, and the two may become paired in memory.[16] Often people with misophonia will report both visual and auditory stimuli that trigger them. I explained to Lisa that she should use the same skills with visual stimuli as those she learned with auditory stimuli. We also talked about practical solutions, such as trying to avert her gaze away from other peoples' mouths. As is true of most people with misophonia, this was difficult for Lisa to do. People with misophonia (or their parents) often ask why a person is compelled to look at something upsetting. In fact, this is one reason a person might appear to be "obsessing" on particular stimuli. A simple explanation based on research[16] often helps family members, teachers, and individuals understand. Again, understanding something often makes it less overwhelming.

6. **Practical solutions**

In addition to helping Lisa understand the underlying mechanisms of misophonia, our interactions guided her to employ practical solutions in her life (e.g., meditation, exercise, texting when in a crowd in order to redirect her attention, using a stress ball, rhythmic entrainment, etc.).

25.7 Additional Question for the Reader

What are the important elements that support teaching coping skills?

- Psychoeducation.
- Learning physiological self-regulation skills.
- Empathic listening and understanding.
- Cognitive reframing.
- Addressing the physiological response.
- Practical solutions.
- Communication with other practitioners.
- Communication with family members (if appropriate).

25.8 Outcome

After 10 weeks, Lisa demonstrated a much clearer understanding of misophonia and how it influenced her daily activities physiologically as well as cognitively and emotionally (the intended effect of psychoeducation). In addition, she was able to separate the idea that people were triggers and came to understand that sounds were the issue and that, for reasons that are not yet known, certain peoples' reaction to sounds may be worse than others. She also utilized her athletic abilities to work on her arousal level by working out with light weights each day in her room. Lisa found this and four-square breathing very helpful "in the moment." On a practical level, she utilized her ear-level sound generators to mask sounds and used her hand gripper to help her system back to homeostasis. She also learned how to explain misophonia to others when necessary. Although her self-confidence and

sense of self-efficacy were not measured, her activity level, interaction with family members, confidence in managing the condition, and her reported sense of greater tolerance to potentially triggering sounds improved substantially from her initial contact.

References

[1] Brout JJ, Edelstein M, Erfanian M, et al. Investigating misophonia: a review of the empirical literature, clinical implications, and a research agenda. Front Neurosci. 2018; 12: 1–13

[2] Cavanna AE, Seri S. Misophonia: current perspectives. Neuropsychiatr Dis Treat. 2015; 11:2117–2123

[3] Meltzer J, Herzfeld M. Tinnitus, hyperacusis, and misophonia toolbox. In: Seminars in hearing, Vol. 35. New York: Thieme Medical Publishers; 2014:121–130

[4] Kisley MA, Noecker TL, Guinther PM. Comparison of sensory gating to mismatch negativity and self-reported perceptual phenomena in healthy adults. Psychophysiology. 2004; 41 (4):604–612

[5] Rosenthal MZ, Neacsiu AD, Geiger PJ, et al. Emotional reactivity to personally-relevant and standardized sounds in borderline personality disorder. Cognit Ther Res. 2016; 40: 314–327

[6] Frank B, McKay D. The suitability of an inhibitory learning approach in exposure when habituation fails: a clinical application to misophonia. Cogn. Behav. Pract. 2019; 26(1): 130–142

[7] Brandon F, Dean McKay, The suitability of an inhibitory learning approach in exposure when habituation fails: a clinical application to misophonia. Cognitive and Behavioral Practice. 2019; 26(1):130–142

[8] Schröder AE, Vulink NC, van Loon AJ, Denys DA. Cognitive behavioral therapy is effective in misophonia: An open trial. J Affect Disord. 2017; 217:289–294

[9] Sukhbinder Kumar, Pradeep Dheerendra, Mercede Erfanian, et al. The Motor Basis for Misophonia. Journal of Neuroscience. 2021 June; 41(26):5762–5770; DOI: https://doi.org/10.1523/JNEUROSCI.0261-21.2021

[10] Webber TA, Johnson PL, Storch EA. Pediatric misophonia with comorbid obsessive-compulsive spectrum disorders. Gen Hosp Psychiatry. 2014; 36(2):231.e1–231.e2

[11] Kumar S, Tansley-Hancock O, Sedley W, et al. The brain basis for misophonia. Curr Biol. 2017; 27(4):527–533

[12] Jastreboff PJ, Jastreboff MM. Treatments for decreased sound tolerance (hyperacusis and misophonia). In: Seminars in hearing, Vol. 35. New York: Thieme Medical Publishers; 2014:105–120

[13] Ben-Sasson A, Carter AS, Briggs-Gowan MJ. The development of sensory over-responsivity from infancy to elementary school. J Abnorm Child Psychol. 2010; 38(8):1193–1202

[14] Van Hulle C, Lemery-Chalfant K, Goldsmith HH. Trajectories of sensory over-responsivity from early to middle childhood: birth and temperament risk factors. PLoS One. 2015; 10(6): e0129968

[15] LeDoux J. Anxious: using the brain to understand and treat fear and anxiety. New York: Penguin; 2015

[16] Schröder A, Vulink N, Denys D. Misophonia: diagnostic criteria for a new psychiatric disorder. PLoS One. 2013; 8(1): e54706

Suggested Readings

Jennifer Jo Brout. Regulate, Reason & Reassure: A Parent's Guide to Understanding and Managing Misophonia

Misophonia Literature Review

Brout JJ, Edelstein M, Erfanian M, et al. Investigating misophonia: a review of the empirical literature, clinical implications, and a research agenda. Front Neurosci. 2018; 12:36. A Consensus Definitition of Misophonia https://www.medrxiv.org/content/10.1101/2021.04.05.21254951v1

Resources for Clinicians

https://misophoniaeducation.com/

Resources for Patients and Research Studies

https://www.misophonia.duke.edu/content/what-misophonia

Basic Processes of the Defensive Motivational System (Neuroscience)

LeDoux J. Anxious: using the brain to understand and treat fear and anxiety. New York: Penguin; 2015

26 A Case of Early Adolescent Misophonia

Ana Rabasco

A 13-year-old female presents with misophonia.

26.1 Clinical History and Description

This patient is a 13-year-old female seen as a participant in a misophonia treatment research study for children. She reported extreme sensitivity to specific sounds but had not yet sought services from an audiologist, neither had she received previous treatment for misophonia. At the initial session, the patient reported that she had a number of friends and was actively involved in multiple extracurricular activities, including musical theater and cheer leading. She also reported that her parents were divorced and that she alternated between her mother and father's homes daily.

The patient reported that her sound sensitivity largely involved chewing, slurping, and breathing sounds and that the sounds were most bothersome when produced by family members, particularly the patient's mother. The patient and her mother described her reaction to these sounds as extreme, including leaving the situation, crying, curling up in a ball, shaking, and covering her ears. The patient noted that she would feel nauseous and "shivery" when she heard triggering sounds. Because of this, the patient would use noise-cancelling headphones during mealtimes with her family and her mother would often eat meals in a separate room. The patient reported that she had experienced sensitivity to the offending sounds for as long as she could remember; however, her sensitivity intensified over the past year.

26.2 Questions for the Reader

1. What additional case history might be pertinent to this case?
2. What psychological treatment approaches are appropriate for this case?
3. What additional factors should be considered during the course of psychological treatment?

26.3 Discussion of Questions for the Reader

1. *What additional case history might be pertinent to this case?*
   It could be helpful to assess for co-occurring

psychological disorders (e.g., anxiety, depression, posttraumatic stress disorder [PTSD]). For example, research has found that PTSD exacerbates the severity of misophonic symptoms.[1] In addition, a family history of misophonia may also be relevant, as one large-scale study on misophonia found that one-third of the sample reported that they had family members with similar sound intolerance, or annoyance hyperacusis symptoms.[1]

2. *What psychological treatment approaches are appropriate for this case?*
   Cognitive behavioral therapy (CBT), with an emphasis on exposure and desensitization, should be considered as a way to facilitate the patient's recognition that trigger sounds produce an emotional response that is disproportionate to the sound's value. While research in this area is extremely limited, several case studies and pilot studies have suggested, based on qualitative findings, that CBT for misophonia is a helpful treatment modality.[2,3]

3. *What additional factors should be considered during the course of psychological treatment?*
   Because intervention necessitates that the patient's parents be involved in the exposure exercises, the dynamics of the patient's relationship with her parents is an important consideration. In addition, the patient's emotional state at each session was taken into account, as her level of fatigue and stress could affect her motivation and ability to tolerate the exposure exercises. Finally, the study protocol required monitoring the patient's compliance with exposure homework and attending treatment sessions in order to identify potential problems, as well as to maximize the benefits of the intervention.

26.4 Final Diagnosis and Recommended Treatment

The patient presented with symptoms consistent with annoyance hyperacusis, or misophonia, at the initial intake session. The patient was enrolled in the study treatment of 12 sessions of CBT for misophonia conducted twice per week (6 weeks total) over webcam with a study therapist. The intervention protocol involved psychoeducation, gradually progressing through an exposure hierarchy, reducing family accommodation for misophonia, and enhancing general distress tolerance. Intervention protocol also included daily exposure homework assigned by the study therapist.

26.5 Outcome

The experimental intervention began with exposure exercises at the bottom of exposure hierarchy generated by the patient and therapist. These exposures consisted of watching 1 to 2 minutes of autonomous sensory meridian response (ASMR) chewing videos on YouTube.com on a low volume. Once the patient was able to tolerate the videos, she began exposure exercises with her family members, such as 2 minutes of her father eating carrots from 10 feet away. Exposure exercise difficulty was gradually increased until the patient reached the top of her exposure hierarchy (her mother chewing in an exaggerated manner right next to her). Throughout this process, the patient did not consistently follow the daily exposure exercises assigned by the study therapist. She typically completed 2 to 3 days of homework a week, rather than the recommended seven. However, despite inconsistent compliance, by the CBT course's conclusion, the patient's misophonia symptoms decreased. For example, she experienced no distress when her father sat next to her chewing in an exaggerated manner (e.g., open-mouthed, extreme smacking) for at least 5 minutes. The patient still experienced self-reported mild distress (subjective unit of distress rating of 20 out of 100) when her mother sat next to her chewing in an exaggerated manner for at least 5 minutes. The patient was able to tolerate family dinners without wearing noise-cancelling headphones with little to no distress. The patient and her parents reported that they felt she no longer experienced functional impairment due to annoyance hyperacusis and that they were satisfied with the intervention outcome. Overall, the patient demonstrated marked improvement in her misophonia symptoms over the course of 6 weeks of CBT.

At the final session, it was recommended that the patient continue with daily exposure exercises to maintain the improvement made during the experimental protocol. In addition, a referral to a nearby therapist who uses CBT as a treatment for misophonia was provided.

26.6 Key Points Self-Efficacy Strategies for Patients

- Misophonia can be successfully managed with CBT that emphasizes exposure, accurate assessment of the trigger sounds, and gradual reduction of the accommodations provided by friends and family.

References

[1] Rouw R, Erfanian M. A large-scale study of misophonia. J Clin Psychol. 2018; 74(3):453–479

[2] Bernstein RE, Angell KL, Dehle C. A brief course of cognitive behavioural therapy for the treatment of misophonia: a case example. Cogn Behav Therap. 2013; 6(E10)

[3] Frank, B., & McKay, D. The suitability of an inhibitory learning approach in exposure when habituation fails: a clinical application to misophonia. Cogn Behav Practice. 2019; 26(1): 130–142

27 Superhero Treatment for Sound Sensitivity

Melissa Karp

27.1 Clinical History and Description

MC, a 14-year-old female, was first seen in the clinic in July, 2017, at which time she reported sound-related difficulties that started months earlier. Trigger sounds were chewing, breathing, and hiccups. Exposure to these sounds resulted in extreme distress, anger, and frustration. MC's sensitivity impaired concentration and sleep as it influenced family dynamics and social/recreational situations. A clinical psychologist diagnosed MC with anxiety and depression linked to the effects of the triggering sounds.

Eating with the family at the dinner table was one of the more disrupted activities and MC was able to pinpoint the specific sounds of each family member that were triggers. She was wearing noise cancelling hearing protection at the dinner table. This strategy was suggested by her psychologist.

When she was exposed to a trigger sound, she exhibited a physical reflex of inhaling and tensing her shoulders and squeezing her hands.

None of the following warning signs of ear disease were noted: visible congenital/traumatic deformity of the ear, history of active drainage from the ear, history of sudden or rapidly progressive hearing loss, acute or chronic dizziness, unilateral hearing loss, an audiometric air-bone gap equal to or greater than 15 dB, evidence of significant cerumen buildup, and/or ear pain or discomfort.[1]

27.2 Audiological Testing

Otoscopy revealed clear ear canals with intact tympanic membranes, bilaterally.

27.2.1 Pure-Tone Testing

Hearing sensitivity was within normal limits bilaterally (see ▶ Fig. 27.1).

27.2.2 Sound Tolerance Testing

Uncomfortable loudness level (UCL) testing was completed and thresholds were obtained from 70 dB HL to 90 dB HL, indicating mild-to-moderate hyperacusis.[2]

27.3 Questionnaires

The Amsterdam Misophonia Scale (A-MISO-S) is an adaptation of the Yale-Brown Obsessive Compulsive Scale (Y-BOCS) and was developed by researchers in Amsterdam.[3] The severity of the misophonia is determined by the sum of the points from the self-completed questionnaire (see the box below). MC scored 17, which is considered severe. She responded to the question, "What would be the worst thing that could happen if you were unable to avoid the misophonic sounds?" by writing, "I could get so angry sometimes, I get the feeling my stomach is turning and it's so frustrating I feel like

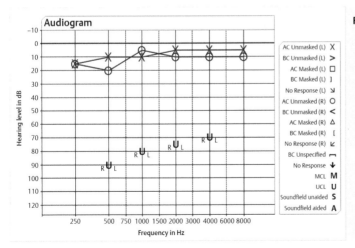

Fig. 27.1 Audiometric test results.

I could hit someone/something and could hurt myself or others." It is important to note that MC does not act on these feelings.

Misophonia Severity (A-MISO-S)

0–4: Subclinical, no treatment needed
5–9: Mild
10–14: Moderate
15–19: Severe
20–24: Extreme

The Misophonia Assessment Questionnaire (MAQ) consists of 21 questions that are scored between 0 and 3 points depending on how often the patient experiences symptoms.[4] This was completed by the patient and her mother. MC scored 48, placing her in the severe category. This is consistent with the A-MISO-S scale.

Misophonia Severity (MAQ)

0–11: Subclinical, no treatment needed
12–24: Mild
25–37: Moderate
38–50: Severe
51–63: Extreme

The Misophonia Coping Responses is a questionnaire that evaluates coping responses to trigger sounds.[5] MC's responses indicate she is experiencing visual triggers (seeing a person eat, for example) in addition to auditory triggers. The phenomenon of visual triggers is explained by the theory that misophonia is a sensory hyper-reactivity syndrome that can shift from typical auditory triggers to a visual trigger.[3] She is in control of her actions in her coping responses.

The Misophonia Emotional Response Questionnaire[6] is a self-completed assessment that asks the patient to rate how often they feel the listed emotional responses to their trigger sound. It is important to note that these responses are what the patient feels and not what actions they take. MC's trigger sounds elicit severe emotional distress—such as hate, anger, rage, disgust, resentment, and despair.

27.4 Questions for the Reader

1. What diagnosis can best be described by this patient?

2. Is this an auditory or psychological diagnosis?
3. What should be recommended regarding the use of hearing protection for this patient?

27.5 Discussion of Questions for the Reader

1. *What diagnosis can best be described by this patient?*
   Misophonia does not appear in the fifth edition of the Diagnostic and Statistical Manual of Mental Disorders (DSM-5) as a discrete disorder. There are arguments to be made for audiologists using the code for "Hyperacusis" or "Abnormal Auditory Perception" although neither quite captures the misophonic patient experience. In this case, hyperacusis (ICD-10 H93.233) was diagnosed.

2. *Is this an auditory or psychological diagnosis?*
   Misophonia, as many other sensory processing disorders, is a as bit of both and appears to occupy a spectrum from mild annoyance to disabling. From an audiological perspective, misophonia involves the auditory pathways and a reaction to what is perceived, similar to tinnitus. From a psychological perspective, misophonia does not require the auditory stimuli to provoke a reaction (such as anger at anticipation of triggers and reaction to visual triggers), and the behaviors that are provoked are in line with "Other Specified Obsessive-Compulsive and Related Disorder." Neurological factors have also been identified that contribute to misophonia, including abnormal activation, functional connections, structural changes in the brain, and enhanced autonomic responses in the body.[7]

3. *What should be recommended regarding the use of hearing protection for this patient?*
   Overuse of hearing protection can result in heightened sensitivity to sound. We recommended having her wear earphones that played pink noise (a sound she preferred over white noise) to ensure the auditory system was receiving stimulation instead of using the noise cancellation feature for quiet.[8] We also had the family enrich the sound environment at the dinner table with music or nature sounds and advised the transition from the hearing protection to the enriched sound environment.

27.6 Final Diagnosis and Recommended Treatment

MC was diagnosed with hyperacusis (H93.233) and misophonia, although no specific diagnosis code exists for the latter. Loudness hyperacusis is a hearing disorder characterized by an increased sensitivity to common sounds (i.e., a collapsed tolerance to usual environmental sound) accompanied by distress and/or avoidance strategies. Annoyance hyperacusis, or misophonia, results from enhanced functional connections between the auditory and limbic and autonomic nervous systems, which may result in a conditioned reflex analogous to a "fight or flight" event.[9] Intervention prioritizes weakening and then abolishing these connections using protocols appropriate for the extinction of conditioned responses. It should be noted that in pure misophonia, auditory sensitivity and loudness tolerances are within normal limits. Due to the mixed nature of MC's diagnosis, intervention targeted the misophonia triggers first and then sought to address any remaining loudness hyperacusis component.

Recommendations included the reduction of hearing protection use and sound therapy to avoid silence and decrease the sensory contrast between the triggers and the ambient noise and reduce the clarity of trigger sounds. This was to be accomplished with nonoccluding devices playing white or pink noise. A protocol to extinguish misophonia by linking currently offensive sounds with positive sounds was provided as well using progressive muscle relaxation exercises.[10] A script was provided to the family to use as a guideline.[11] The family was counseled to keep the lines of communication open should MC become overwhelmed or no longer able to not act on her feelings of self-harm or harm to others that immediate psychological intervention would be necessary. The family was working with a psychologist and expressed understanding of the importance of monitoring MC for these concerns.

27.7 Outcome

Sound generators and therapy recommendations were initially rejected by MC and she was lost to follow-up for 16 months, finally returning to the clinic in November, 2016. Follow-up in November 2018 was completed. MC and her family had tried cognitive behavioral therapy (CBT) after MC displayed self-harming behaviors that she indicated were related to the distress produced by triggering sounds. Eventually, she was removed from public school and was being home schooled as she could not tolerate the trigger sounds in the school environment. She would only eat in her room and was not able to be present if anyone in the family was chewing or eating. Acupuncture and chiropractic care were also tried with no success. After doing Internet research, the family decided to return to the clinic and try the recommendations again.

Intervention was based on the Jastreboff protocol 4 for treatment of sound sensitivity.[8] MC is a Marvel movie fan and had been unable to go to the movies due to potential of being triggered by attendees eating snacks at the theater. We opted to use Marvel movies as a positive stimulus in a desensitization approach to pair with negative trigger sounds. She used her smartphone and recorded a family member eating. While watching the Marvel movies, she would glance at the recording for a few seconds and then put the phone down and continue watching the movie. When that was not bothersome, she turned up the volume of the triggering sound gradually. When that was not bothersome, she had that family member sit in the room with her and eat in short controlled bursts whose timing MC could control and then ultimately eat at will. MC took control of this task and became interested in researching and filming a documentary about misophonia to educate others. She wore the sound generators and was able to return to school part time and continue home school part time with the intent of transitioning to a full-time public-school attendance. Her parents reported that, more often than not, she is able to sit at the dinner table for at least part of the meal without distress.

Follow-up in February 2019 revealed A-MISO-S score at 10, MAQ at 25, Misophonia Coping Response revealed visual triggers were no longer an issue, and Misophonia Emotional Response Questionnaire yielded less emotional distress than previously reported. Treatment is ongoing (▶ Fig. 27.2 and ▶ Fig. 27.3).

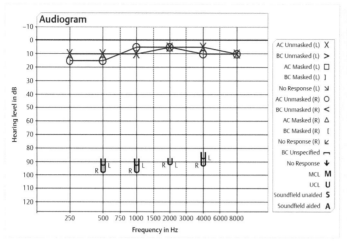

Fig. 27.2 Follow-up audiometric testing demonstrating improvement, compared to ▶ Fig. 27.1, in uncomfortable loudness levels (U) following intervention.

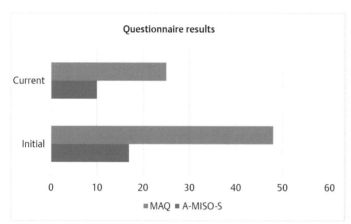

Fig. 27.3 Pre- and postintervention questionnaire results. (MAQ, Misophonia Assessment Questionnaire; A-MISO-S, Amsterdam Misophonia Scale.)

References

[1] American Academy of Otolaryngology-Head and Neck Surgery. Position statement: red flags-warning of ear disease; 2019. [online] https://www.entnet.org/content/position-statement-red-flags-warning-ear-disease Accessed February 25, 2019

[2] Goldstein B, Shulman A. Tinnitus: hyperacusis and the loudness discomfort level test: a preliminary report. Int Tinnitus J. 1996; 2(1):83–89

[3] Schröder A, Vulink N, Denys D. Misophonia: diagnostic criteria for a new psychiatric disorder. PLoS One. 2013; 8(1): e54706

[4] Johnson M, Dozier T. Misophonia Assessment Questionnaire; MAQ. https://misophoniatreatment.com/wp-content/uploads/2016/02/Binder_all_forms.pdf. Accessed February 21, 2019

[5] Dozier T. Misophonia coping responses. https://misophoniatreatment.com/wp-content/uploads/2016/02/Binder_all_forms.pdf. Accessed February 21, 2019

[6] Dozier T. Misophonia emotional responses. https://misophoniatreatment.com/wp-content/uploads/2016/02/Binder_all_forms.pdf. Accessed February 21, 2019

[7] Kumar S, Tansley-Hancock O, Sedley W, et al. The brain basis for misophonia. Curr Biol. 2017; 27(4):527–533

[8] Jastreboff P, Jastreboff M. Treatments for decreased sound tolerance (hyperacusis and misophonia). Semin Hear. 2014; 35(02):105–120

[9] Tyler RS, Pienkowski M, Roncancio ER, et al. A review of hyperacusis and future directions: part I. Definitions and manifestations. Am J Audiol. 2014; 23(4):402–419. Accessed February 25, 2019

[10] Dozier TH. Understanding and overcoming misophonia: a conditioned aversive reflex disorder. Livermore, CA: Misophonia Treatment Institute; 2017

[11] Bourne E. The anxiety & phobia workbook. 5th ed. Oakland: New Harbinger Publications; 2010

Suggested Readings

Brout JJ, Edelstein M, Erfanian M, et al. Investigating misophonia: a review of the empirical literature, clinical implications, and a research agenda. Front Neurosci. 2018; 12:36

Cutter M. Chomp. Slurp. Smack. SNAP! ASHA Lead. 2018; 23(7):44

Taylor S. Misophonia: a new mental disorder? Med Hypotheses. 2017; 103:109–117

Tinnitus Home Page. (n.d.). Retrieved February 13, 2019, from http://tinnitus-pjj.com/

Section C: Additional Considerations

28 Normal Hearing

Marc Fagelson and Suzanne H. Kimball

One of this text's recurring themes emerges through cases in which patients reporting sound-provoked distress present in the clinic with normal puretone (250–8,000 Hz) audiograms. The situation is not unfamiliar: a person has normal hearing thresholds accompanied by bothersome tinnitus and/or sound intolerance; do they have normal hearing? Such findings should not produce much of a conundrum: no, they do not have normal hearing; they have bothersome symptoms associated with the auditory system that reduce quality of life and influence their ability to function. Yet patients in that situation are told, routinely, that their hearing is normal. The audiogram does not talk, it informs. The practitioner is charged with the accurate interpretation of results for the patient. This text attempts to capture the idea that a normal audiogram often coexists with damage to the mechanisms, namely, hair cells, synapses, neurons, and tracts—the broken piano keys—essential for audition, but whose integrity may not be detectable on the audiogram.

Some of the mechanisms responsible for the tinnitus and sound intolerance symptoms may be triggered by natural compensatory adjustments at a variety of loci along the auditory pathway in response to changes, often difficult to detect, in the integrity of the peripheral system.[1,2] Central compensation may be thought of as increasing auditory gain, decreasing inhibitory processes, or a combination of the two. These mechanisms may unmask pre-existing spontaneous neural activity, thereby producing tinnitus.[3] The central compensation may also produce the unexpected, paradoxical finding that individuals with decreased sensitivity experience uncomfortable loudness at sound levels that individuals with *better* hearing can tolerate easily.[4] That is to say, a symptom of degraded function, regardless of threshold level, may appear as a decreased tolerance for routine, everyday sounds. Patients thus affected may have, simultaneously, hearing loss and decreased loudness tolerance. The impact on dynamic range can be catastrophic. Therefore, it is possible that undetectable peripheral dysfunction provokes central compensation that changes sound perception, specifically by biasing the physical and psychological processing of sound, producing unusually vigorous responses.

"Hidden hearing loss" is one of many terms used when patients with many specific and common complaints related to their ability to communicate may have puretone thresholds in the normal range. Probably all hearing healthcare providers struggled at one time or another with the counseling and intervention options when patients report sound-related challenges despite displaying normal sensitivity. The objective of this brief chapter is not to denigrate the audiogram, but rather to highlight the value of accurate and reasonable interpretation of its findings in challenging cases. As recently as 2013, the durable and prevailing opinion among audiologists likely approached, "No matter how we view the audiogram, even with its known limitations, it is considered the 'gold standard' for audiological diagnosis."[5] Given the aforementioned discrepancy between normal thresholds and a patient profoundly challenged by sound, its status as "gold standard" warrants concern unless that seems too strong.

Perhaps one way to think about audiogram interpretation is to compare the audiogram to something else with which we are familiar, the Snellen eye chart. Clearly, a person with 20/20 vision can perform the task of identifying letters and objects on an eye chart in the clinical setting. However, the same person may experience night blindness, have peripheral field-of-vision problems, contrast insensitivity, or extreme glare sensitivity that would not be captured by the assessment yielding a 20/20 result.[6] Similarly, normal audiograms may accompany impaired words-in-noise recognition, myriad forms of sound intolerance, and severely intrusive tinnitus. Patients may experience additional difficulty accessing resources or care if they perform well when speech in noise or loudness tolerance is tested. But healthcare providers must be cautious; some patients struggle in most environments despite scoring well on speech-in-noise tests, while others can tolerate narrow bands of noise in the clinic at high levels without discomfort despite experiencing sudden and profound rage at hearing a family member eat. Such possibilities merely demonstrate that valid tests do not always capture their intended targets; mostly, we accept this notion. The tests do not lack value, but opportunities to practice their interpretation and integration must be provided to students and practitioners, particularly if audiologists are to formulate and practice management protocols required by the affected patients.

28.1 Questions for the Reader

1. What tests are most important to consider adding to the audiologic evaluation when hidden hearing loss is suspected?
2. Is it correct to provide hearing protection to all patients with sound tolerance issues?

28.2 Discussion of Questions for the Reader

1. *What tests are most important to consider adding to the audiologic evaluation when hidden hearing loss is suspected?*
   Speech-in-noise, extended high-frequency puretone, and loudness tolerance testing are acknowledged as important, not only in this application, but also with regard to hearing aid selection and counseling as well. Several speech-in-noise test instruments are available for clinical use. The value of loudness assessment is less clear; although test results may identify levels at which a patient experiences discomfort, testing loudness tolerance in distressed patients may not be reasonable. It is unfortunate that audiologists lack assessments that target function at the high (tolerance) end of the dynamic range as well as they assess function at the low (threshold) end. Loudness perception test results may vary considerably from trial to trial, showing far more variability than would be found with a validated questionnaire. The Multiple-Activity Scale for Hyperacusis (MASH)[7] and Inventory of Hyperacusis Symptoms (IHS)[8] provide the patients the means by which they can report sound-related problems using instruments whose results are interpreted relative to large numbers of similarly affected individuals. Extended high-frequency threshold testing may require additional equipment; however, its inclusion facilitates interpretation of ototoxicity and noise effects.
2. *Is it correct to provide hearing protection to all patients with sound tolerance issues?*
   Patients experiencing discomfort in the presence of offending sounds may want to employ hearing protection in those instances. Intuitively, this is a good idea—sound bothers

the patient, and in response, the patient uses hearing protection. Unfortunately, the use of protectors may have the unintended effect of *increasing* the neural activity in the central pathways associated with the symptoms of discomfort. Patients can always take along hearing protectors when they anticipate situations that might be uncomfortable, and use the devices only when necessary. Encouraging a patient to minimize use of protectors must be balanced against the possibility of a setback caused by an overexposure; nobody is expected to be a hero and desensitization is more marathon than sprint.

While 10 to 15% of the general population reports tinnitus, nearly 50% of those individuals also experience sound intolerance to some degree.[9,10] Sound therapy can be used as a way to interact with the offending sound (to mask partially or fully), or it can be used as part of a desensitization protocol to tolerate louder increments of sound each day. As many patients with normal hearing have been dissatisfied with the advice, or the lack thereof, from other healthcare professionals, audiologists specializing in tinnitus and sound sensitivities should be equipped to offer some form of rehabilitative help for such individuals. We offer a few suggestions here.

The healthcare provider must be prepared to address patient strategies that, while intuitive, are counterproductive. Desensitization and enrichment[11] with sound may appear the more daunting proposition, but for many patients, compared to their experience of withdrawing from sound, this road less taken may make all the difference. It is our responsibility to steer patients in the direction that may seem the more daunting, but which offers the most reasonable path to a positive outcome. Desensitization requires stimulation, and the effectiveness of hearing aids and masking apps now offer patients options and control over their choice(s) of sound(s) that they need to support strategies intended to reduce powerful aversive reactions to sound.

Dozens of free smartphone applications available in the IOS or Google platforms offer sound therapy sound files in a variety of forms from nature sounds to white noise and everything in between. Basic sound therapy principles and their rationales can be described to the patient, and value of different strategies—total versus partial, or energetic versus informational masking—should guide the choice of therapeutic sound. Patients should employ the sound therapy binaurally using headphones or earbuds to provide either tinnitus masking or desensitizing sound. A bedside speaker or sleep headband can be used at night if the patient experiences sleep disturbance due to tinnitus symptoms. For many patients, education regarding how and why tinnitus and sound intolerance occur, coupled with the use of a sound therapy app, is a cost effective and oftentimes a successful way to reduce bothersome auditory symptoms.

Another option, particularly in instances when earbuds/headphones are impractical for everyday use, is essential/basic level hearing aid technology. Although this option is certainly more expensive for the patient, many of these products can be retailed in the $1,000 to $2,000 range quite easily. This is generally an out-of-pocket expense for the patient, as no hearing loss diagnostic code exists to utilize insurance benefits in most cases. As long as the hearing aids have tinnitus sound generation (TSG) or Bluetooth streaming as an option, any low-gain, basic/essential product can be used. Smartphone compatibility is advised as well in order to take advantage of the use of the aforementioned apps. Turning the hearing aid microphones off and using the TSG as the program setting is optimal for many patients. Some patients do well with the hearing aid microphones turned on with little to no gain provided just so there is an additional enriched sound environment which helps to interact with the tinnitus perception. Smartphone compatibility provides the patient the flexibility to increase or decrease the sound therapy volume throughout the day as indicated. It is vital to give patients the ability to adjust the sound therapy volume. For the patient who does not own a smartphone, a remote control can be purchased along with the hearing aids.

Unfortunately, in this area of practice, it is likely that there are about as many cases that are exceptions as there are cases that follow the rules. The heterogeneity of tinnitus causes, mechanisms, sounds, and effects cannot be unrelated to the fact that although tinnitus can be managed, in most cases, it cannot be shut off. Similarly, disorders of sound tolerance may involve unusual perceptions of loudness, annoyance, fear, pain, and impaired speech recognition in adverse listening conditions.[12,13] The poor correlations between severity of patients' experiences and their audiometric results complicates management and audiologic practice. Do we respond with vigor to patient complaints that we cannot objectively measure, or do we rely solely upon validated clinical protocols that experience tells us do not always capture important elements of patient narratives? For comparison, it is worth considering what healthcare providers do if a patient reports chronic, debilitating headaches when all available objective assessments contraindicate presence of substantial pathology. The healthcare providers would strive to manage the symptom with the understanding that they may not be able to cure the underlying condition causing the headache. Audiologists face similar challenges, particularly when working with patients experiencing bothersome auditory symptoms. Patients with sound intolerance and tinnitus are probably far more common than audiologists care to admit. The vision and flexibility required of audiologists will remain substantial and essential; many of these patients may be hidden in plain sight because their situations are not thoroughly grasped, nor their needs reasonably met. Ultimately, professionals can foster clinical interventions that provide ample opportunity for both patients and healthcare providers to learn from, and to teach each other.

References

[1] Kujawa SG, Liberman MC. Synaptopathy in the noise-exposed and aging cochlea: primary neural degeneration in acquired sensorineural hearing loss. Hear Res. 2015; 330 Pt B:191–199

[2] Eggermont JJ. Effects of long-term non-traumatic noise exposure on the adult central auditory system. Hearing problems without hearing loss. Hear Res. 2017; 352:12–22

[3] Schaette R, McAlpine D. Tinnitus with a normal audiogram: physiological evidence for hidden hearing loss and computational model. J Neurosci. 2011; 31(38):13452–13457

[4] Roberts LE, Sanchez TG, Bruce IC. Tinnitus and hyperacusis: relationship, mechanisms and initiating conditions. In: Fagelson M, Baguley D, eds. Hyperacusis and Disorders of Sound Intolerance: Clinical and Research Perspectives. San Diego, CA: Plural Publishing; 2018

[5] Jerger J. Why the audiogram is upside-down. Int J Audiol. 2013; 52(3):146–150

[6] Ciuffreda KJ, Kapoor N, Rutner D, Suchoff IB, Han ME, Craig S. Occurrence of oculomotor dysfunctions in acquired brain injury: a retrospective analysis. Optometry. 2007; 78 (4):155–161

[7] Dauman R, Bouscau-Faure F. Assessment and amelioration of hyperacusis in tinnitus patients. Acta Otolaryngol. 2005; 125 (5):503–509

[8] Greenberg B, Carlos M. Psychometric properties and factor structure of a new scale to measure hyperacusis: introducing the inventory of hyperacusis symptoms. Ear Hear. 2018; 39 (5):1025–1034

[9] Shargorodsky J, Curhan GC, Farwell WR. Prevalence and characteristics of tinnitus among US adults. Am J Med. 2010; 123(8):711–718

[10] Baguley DM. The epidemiology and natural history of disorders of loudness perception. In: Fagelson M, Baguley D, eds. Hyperacusis and Disorders of Sound Intolerance: Clinical and Research Perspectives. San Diego, CA: Plural Publishing; 2018

[11] Formby C, Hawley ML, Sherlock LP, et al. A sound therapy-based intervention to expand the auditory dynamic range for loudness among persons with sensorineural hearing losses: a randomized placebo-controlled clinical trial. Semin Hear. 2015; 36(2):77–110

[12] Tyler RS, Pienkowski M, Roncancio ER, et al. A review of hyperacusis and future directions: part I. Definitions and manifestations. Am J Audiol. 2014; 23(4):402–419

[13] Theodoroff SM, Reavis KM, Griest SE, Carlson KF, Hammill TL, Henry JA. Decreased sound tolerance associated with blast exposure. Sci Rep. 2019; 9(1):10204

29 Tinnitus and CoVID-19

Suzanne H. Kimball and Marc Fagelson

29.1 Simulated Case

While much is still unknown about the lingering health effects of CoVID-19, in the past year many audiologists reported patients experiencing otologic symptoms that reportedly appeared after a positive CoVID-19 diagnosis. The editors of this book thought it important to include a chapter on the presence of emerging and lingering tinnitus symptoms in patients diagnosed with CoVID-19.

29.2 History

RMK is a 48-year-old female seen in our clinic in early 2021. RMK was diagnosed with CoVID-19 via a nasal swab in November 2020. Anosmia, or loss of the sense of smell, was the only CoVID-19 symptom she reported. RMK exhibited significant anxiety regarding her diagnosis, as she expressed apprehension concerning the lack of conclusive data regarding the long-term health effects of CoVID-19 and/or the lingering side effects, particularly a permanent loss of smell. On this date, RMK reported left-sided, unilateral tinnitus with onset immediately following her CoVID-19 diagnosis. RMK had no complaints of hearing loss or other otologic symptoms.

29.3 Audiometric Test Results

RMK completed the Tinnitus Handicap Inventory (THI)[1] and the Tinnitus Functional Index (TFI)[2] prior to presenting in our clinic. She scored a 72 on the THI and 84 on the TFI indicating severely bothersome tinnitus that affected many aspects of her life. RMK reported that she had not received any type of hearing testing/screening since grade school.

RMK completed a full audiometric and tinnitus evaluation. She was visibly anxious throughout the test procedures, but overall her reliability was considered excellent. Immittance testing yielded bilateral type A tympanograms. Pure-tone test results indicated a bilateral, mild, sensorineural hearing loss at 4,000 Hz and above. Speech recognition thresholds (SRTs) were established at 25 dB HL bilaterally. Word recognition testing yielded scores of 96% correct at 55 dB HL for both ears in quiet. Acoustic reflex thresholds were not obtained out

of concern that testing would exacerbate her tinnitus symptoms.

Loudness tolerance levels were obtained after the basic audiologic evaluation, and were within normal limits for both ears for both speech and pure-tone stimuli (greater than 90 dB HL).[3] High-frequency audiometry indicated a mild-to-moderate hearing loss from 9 kHz through 16 kHz with no measurable thresholds beyond that frequency. A tinnitus evaluation including pitch match, loudness match, minimal masking (MML) for wideband and narrowband noise, and residual inhibition was completed. She demonstrated partial residual inhibition for 35 seconds following presentation of a white noise for 1 minute at 10 dB SL re: MML.

29.4 Questions for the Reader

1. Does CoVID-19 cause tinnitus symptoms?
2. What other tests could be utilized with this patient?
3. What are the possible management options for this patient?

29.5 Discussion of Questions for the Reader

1. *Does CoVID-19 cause tinnitus symptoms?*
   It has long been established that hearing loss can result from viruses such a cytomegalovirus (CMV), maternal rubella, measles, mumps, and meningitis.[4,5] In addition, conditions such as auditory neuropathy have been shown in patients with Guillain-Barre syndrome, which is known to be associated with a coronavirus.[4] According to Almufarrij et al,[6] auditory neuropathy could be an adverse effect of CoVID-19, as the coronavirus is known to cause peripheral neuropathy, including sensory neuropathy. Almufarrij and colleagues[6] conducted a rapid systematic review and concluded that otologic symptoms such as hearing loss, tinnitus, and vertigo were reported among a small percentage of CoVID-19 patients; however, many of the studies reviewed were considered of poor quality with significant flaws in research design. In a follow-up study at 1 year post the onset of the global

pandemic, Almufarrij and colleagues concluded that tinnitus was reported in approximately 15% of CoVID-19 patients, about double the percentage of hearing loss (8%) and vertigo (7%). The researchers concluded, however, that the haste in which many publications were made available in such a short amount of time suggested readers should exercise caution when drawing conclusions regarding CoVID-19 prevalence and symptom reporting. In particular, a change in status of otologic symptoms prior to a CoVID-19 diagnosis went unreported in many of the studies.

2. *What other tests could be utilized with this patient?*
   As with any tinnitus patient that presents with high levels of anxiety and/or depression, a screening tool such as the Hospital Anxiety and Depression Scale (HADS)[7] could be used to determine if a referral to a mental health profession may be in order. Decades of literature linking high levels of anxiety and depression in patients with debilitating tinnitus have been established.[8]

3. *What are the possible management options for this patient?*
   Amplification with concurrent sound therapy (combination device) could be helpful for this patient to provide a sound-enriched environment. If hearing aids are not desired, standalone sound therapy devices (i.e., tinnitus maskers, hearing aids with masking circuitry and low- or no acoustic gain, a sound therapy app on a smartphone with the use of earbuds/headphones) could be utilized.

29.6 Recommendations and Outcomes

Binaural amplification was recommended for this patient; however, due to budget constraints the patient did not move forward with the purchase of hearing aids. She was counseled regarding the use of sound therapy presented through a smartphone app. She was instructed to set the sound therapy (of her choice, white noise, environmental sounds, etc., as found on the app) at a volume level so that she perceived both the app sound and her tinnitus. She was counseled to employ sound whenever her tinnitus was most bothersome to her throughout her day. The patient was encouraged to return to the clinic in 6 months or sooner if her symptoms persisted as well as to practice relaxation techniques

such as Mindfulness Based Tinnitus Stress Reduction (MBTSR).[9,10] In addition, the patient was counseled regarding referral to a mental health professional to address her anxiety and depression symptoms.

29.7 Self-Efficacy for the Clinician

Otologic symptoms such as hearing loss, vertigo, and particularly tinnitus have been reported in patients positively identified with CoVID-19 since the global pandemic began in late 2019/early 2020. According to Almufarrij et al,[6] these symptoms might be due to one of the following three factors: (1) direct viral infections of the inner ear or the auditory nerve; (2) autoimmune attack by antibodies or immune cells, or damage caused by excessive production of cytokines, which cause inflammation; or (3) blood clots that block the blood supply to the cochlea or semicircular canals which deprives them of oxygen. While prevalence data may be overestimated at this point,[6] the chance that audiologists will continue to see post-CoVID-19 tinnitus patients is highly likely. Beukes et al[11] additionally support this claim; as in their study, a small percentage of participants reported initial onset or exacerbated existing tinnitus post CoVID-19 diagnosis. Anxiety and depression regarding the tinnitus *and* post CoVID-19 symptoms should not be overlooked. Screening tools should be employed, and referral to mental health professionals is warranted as necessary. Drawing conclusions regarding tinnitus being caused by CoVID-19 remains somewhat speculative. With this case study, it is unknown if the patient's hearing loss was preexisting prior to her CoVID-19 diagnosis; therefore, auditory damage may have been present prior to contracting CoVID-19. Her tinnitus symptoms may have developed due to her increased anxiety regarding her coronavirus diagnosis which may be the case with many patients in the future.

References

[1] Newman CW, Jacobson GP, Spitzer JB. Development of the Tinnitus Handicap Inventory. Arch Otolaryngol Head Neck Surg. 1996; 122(2):143–148

[2] Meikle MB, Henry JA, Griest SE, et al. The tinnitus functional index: development of a new clinical measure for chronic, intrusive tinnitus. Ear Hear. 2012; 33(2):153–176

[3] Sherlock LP, Formby C. Estimates of loudness, loudness discomfort, and the auditory dynamic range: normative estimates, comparison of procedures, and test-retest reliability. J Am Acad Audiol. 2005; 16(2):85–100

[4] Munro KJ, Uus K, Almufarrij I, Chaudhuri N, Yioe V. Persistent self-reported changes in hearing and tinnitus in post-hospitalisation COVID-19 cases. Int J Audiol. 2020; 59(12): 889–890

[5] Young YH. Contemporary review of the causes and differential diagnosis of sudden sensorineural hearing loss. Int J Audiol. 2020; 59(4):243–253

[6] Almufarrij I, Uus K, Munro KJ. Does coronavirus affect the audio-vestibular system? A rapid systematic review. Int J Audiol. 2020; 59(7):487–491

[7] Zigmond AS, Snaith RP. The hospital anxiety and depression scale. Acta Psychiatr Scand. 1983; 67(6):361–370

[8] Bhatt JM, Bhattacharyya N, Lin HW. Relationships between tinnitus and the prevalence of anxiety and depression. Laryngoscope. 2017; 127(2):466–469

[9] Gans JJ, O'Sullivan P, Bircheff V. Mindfulness based tinnitus stress reduction pilot study. Mindfulness. 2012; 3(4)

[10] Philippot P, Nef F, Clauw L, de Romrée M, Segal Z. A randomized controlled trial of mindfulness-based cognitive therapy for treating tinnitus. Clin Psychol Psychother. 2012; 19(5):411–419

[11] Beukes EW, Baguley DM, Jacquemin L, et al. Changes in tinnitus experiences during the COVID-19 pandemic. Front Public Health. 2020; 8:592878

Index

Note: Page numbers set **bold** or *italic* indicate headings or figures, respectively.